DEAR
DiARY,
DOES THIS
CANCER
MAKE
MY ASS
LOOK FAT?

DEAR DIARY,

DOES THIS
CANCER
MAKE
MY ASS
LOOK FAT?

A HEARTFELT MEMOIR
WITH A PINCH OF SARCASM

KIMBERLY TRONIC

ATOMIC TANGO

Printed in the United States of America

Book Design by Jane Frey
Photography by Chris Panagakis
Edited by John DeDakis
Illustrations by Roman Ya/Shutterstock

ISBN-13: 978-1-7336086-0-2

Atomic Tango Publishing
www.AtomicTango.com

For Jon

For everyone at Cedars Sinai, who supported me both physically and emotionally

For Dr. Andrew Li, the best oncologist on planet earth

For my family

And for my kindred spirits battling The Big C

CONTENTS

INTRODUCTION

IMAGINE WAKING UP and hearing, "You have cancer."

The first words I want to hear in the morning are, "Would you like a large coffee, or an extra extra extra large coffee?" I'm not in a mindset to deal with news about my health. Especially not news of this caliber. And especially not news that I'm totally, thoroughly, and unequivocally unprepared for.

It's funny how three simple words can monumentally impact your life. That teeny little phrase, which takes only a moment to say, unleashes a tsunami of feelings, and instantly changes everything forever.

Even worse than getting the actual news was getting the news before my morning coffee. I would've been better equipped for the C-bomb had it gone like this:

Woman: Hey, Kim. Here's your venti iced coffee with almond milk and stevia. I added the extra ice you asked for, too.

Me: Awesome, thanks!

Woman: No problem. Oh, I meant tell you....You have ovarian cancer.

Me: Really? That sucks. Did you also remember my reduced fat turkey bacon sandwich?

But that's not how it went down. I had no coffee, no breakfast sandwich, and no quippy reply.

I don't think anyone is ever prepared to hear the news. Once the C-bomb is detonated, you're thrust into an alternate universe, forced to face shit and handle situations you never anticipated.

Everyone has his/her own coping mechanisms. Mine turned out to be a mixture of laughter, weird costumes, bright wigs, journaling, and spending hundreds of dollars on watermelon. I discovered that maintaining a sense of humor allowed me to battle this scary shit storm with a smile (most of the time).

My patience was tested, my dignity was stripped away, and my strength took a beating. I truly got my ass kicked. But I unearthed a whole fresh layer of resolve and pushed through seemingly insurmountable obstacles every day.

I hope you enjoy reading my story as much as I enjoyed living it. Well, actually, I fucking hated living it, but shut up and keep reading.

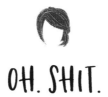

PART ONE

OH. SHIT.

Friday, January 27, 2017 | Los Angeles

I've been unpacking all day. Yesterday I returned from Boston, where I got to see my parents. They are my world. I'd been bummed I didn't get to see them over Christmas, so having a solid week to bask in their love and humor (and home cooked meals and free laundry) was an absolute treat.

Met up with Elina for lunch. It's kinda nice being unemployed (ahem, I mean it's nice being a freelance writer) and having the freedom to chill with friends on a weekday afternoon. Was great catching up with her. I love Elina's magnetic energy and ability to laugh at everything. I told her about this weird pain in my upper right abdomen. The pain has been off-and-on for the last couple of months, and it bothered me during lunch. She said she sometimes gets a pain like that too and figures it's stress or indigestion.

Maybe it's stress from indigestion because I eat too much hot sauce?

———

Friday, February 3, 2017

OK, this whole freelance thing is starting to bother me. I need a full-time job. I'm an extrovert and need human energy around me.

And that stupid stomach pain disappeared for a few days, but it's back again. What the hell is causing it? I think my liver is in that area.

Oh crap. I knew I shouldn't have drunk so much Goldschläger in college. That shit is poison and now my liver is failing me at the tender age of thirty-six. How long does it take to get on the liver transplant list? Isn't there a national shortage or something? Maybe I'm thinking of helium.

Thursday, February 9, 2017

OMG. My friend called with a job opportunity! He's the CMO at a tech startup and needs a Marketing Manager to work under him. He basically offered me the job and said to come in Monday so I can meet their CEO. If all goes well, the job is mine!

Byeeeee, ~~unemployment~~ freelancing—2017 for the win!

Monday, February 13, 2017

Spent the entire weekend putting outfits together and practicing my best "Hire Me" spiel. Was incredibly nervous this morning, but reminded myself that Jake (the CMO) must think I'm qualified. Seemed like the interview went well. I mostly felt confident, but they asked about a couple of things I don't know about, like analytics and Photoshop. I was honest about my skills and lack thereof. I tried to convey that I'm a quick learner and eager to broaden my expertise. We'll see what happens.

I was thankful they didn't pull that, "Where do you see yourself in five years?" stuff. I never know what to say. Part of me wants to chime in with, "Well, honestly, Simon, I envision a future where every morning I wake up, and a hunky, shirtless fireman gives me a fresh almond milk latte while I spread out on my purple velvet couch with eighteen cats while binge-watching *The Real Housewives of Orange County*."

Tuesday, February 14, 2017

What an awesome way to celebrate Valentine's Day. I got the job, and I start next week! The salary is lower than I would have liked, but if I stick with the company and prove my value, I know it will increase over time. Also, that stupid pain in my stomach is back. I think I should get it checked out. Now that I'll have good insurance at the job, I can afford a liver replacement. Plus, having a new liver means I can abuse it without any repercussions. Which is perfect, because this weekend will contain major champagne toasts.

Cheers to me!

Tuesday, February 21, 2017

First day of work. Holy moly, I love my job. It's great to wake up in the morning with a purpose. To be surrounded by other bright-eyed, creative people. To indulge in watercooler chitchat. (OK, there's actually no watercooler, but we can talk by the kitchen sink.) I can't wait to participate in meetings and use Post-its and sniff all the whiteboard markers.

The office is a huge, beautiful, open coworking space with incredible ambiance. The building is decked out like a camp cabin, with dark wood everywhere and photo-real forest wallpaper adorning the conference rooms. The lobby has puzzles and checkers scattered throughout, and a huge picnic table monopolizes the kitchen area.

My bosses rock. The CEO and COO gave me a warm, friendly welcome and invited me to a group lunch. I immediately felt at ease and our conversation flowed seamlessly. I'm thrilled to be part of this team.

Wednesday, March 1, 2017

OK, WTF is going on with my stomach?

I went to Urgent Care this morning and they think it's my gall-bladder. *Congratulations, liver, you're off the hook!* The doctor took my blood and poked around my belly and asked a bunch of questions. She suspects I passed a gallbladder stone, which would account for the discomfort. She told me to avoid fatty foods since those can trigger gallbladder issues. Fine with me. I probably should drop ~~ten~~ twenty pounds anyway.

Thursday, March 9, 2017

The Urgent Care doctor said they'd call if they found anything alarming, but I didn't hear back, so I guess nothing's wrong. OK, gallbladder, please behave and I promise not to send too much fried chicken your way. Spent awhile Googling gallbladder issues and the photos freaked me out.

Note to self: stay away from WebMD.

I have a sneaking suspicion that WebMD was created by companies that make anti-anxiety medication, because any time I use the site, I'm absolutely certain I caught mono, leprosy, swine flu, chicken pox, and scarlet fever.

Wednesday, March 15, 2017

Have I mentioned I love my job? Jake is a dream to work for. He doesn't micromanage and trusts me to get things done. And I feel comfortable asking for help when I need it. I'm so lucky! I get to write, play on social media, brainstorm, and contribute to marketing campaigns. Plus, I adore the people around me. Our intern is basically a mini-me (except she's skinnier, smarter, taller, more graceful, and a million times prettier, but other than that, we're identical twins). And I discovered the woman a few desks over is a literary agent. (That explains the piles of books on her desk.) We've started making small talk (mostly about my diverse necklace collection) and she's sweet. I might pick her brain about self-publishing since I've been working on a collection of essays since 2013 and I hope to self-publish through Amazon. I bet she'll have some solid advice.

———————

Monday, March 20, 2017

OMG. Today I chatted with Jill, the literary agent, and I can't believe this, but she signed me as a client! I'm shocked. When I inquired about self-publishing, she explained how it works and wanted to know why I asked. She liked my concept and requested a writing sample. I emailed her the first essay, and I kept (not-so) discreetly glancing over to see if she laughed or smiled. Later in the afternoon I casually strolled over to see what she thought and she offered to sign me on the spot.

"You're a great writer and this is hilarious. I can't guarantee anything, but let's do this!" she said.

I stared at her with wide eyes and mouth agape, like a doofus. Mind. Fucking. Blown. This is the best news I've ever gotten.

I knew this would be a good year!

———————

Tuesday, March 28, 2017

After a week of pretending I understand legal jargon, I signed Jill's contract. *I officially have a literary agent.* That's a statement I never thought I would say. I'm still in awe that I might actually be a published author one day. I want to email my high school English teacher and say, "Look at me, Ms. Matasso. How do you feel about that C+ now?"

On top of that, with each passing week, I increasingly love my job. Startups are sometimes chaotic since you wear dozens of different hats, but that appeals to my ADD-riddled mind. I want to stay here for a long time.

To celebrate the new job and literary contract, I'm treating myself to a new tattoo. It's gonna cover most of my upper arm and Mom will hate it because she thinks tattoos are trashy. I won't tell her until it's done because I don't want her to ground me, or give me that awful, "I'm not mad, I'm just disappointed" spiel which completely wrecks my emotional well-being. But #YOLO.

Monday, April 3, 2017

Blechhhh. I felt nauseated all day. Not bad enough that I had my head over a toilet, but enough that food repulsed me. Some dude heated up Indian food in the kitchen and it may as well have been a Tupperware of dog feces. Could this be a flu? Did I eat some spoiled lettuce?

Tuesday, April 4, 2017

Still queasy today. *Uh oh, could I be preggo?* That would suck. All my life I've been adamant about not wanting kids, but I experienced a mental shift once I turned thirty-six. I still don't necessarily want a child now, but maybe someday. *Would I have the stomach for an abortion?* I honestly don't know. I'm certainly not ready to care for a small human—I can hardly take care of myself. I use my hamper as a dinner table. I use socks for napkins. I still don't know how to use my oven. I don't own an umbrella, or an iron, or curtains. And I'll never fucking understand what "escrow" means.

Wednesday, April 5, 2017

Oh God. Queasy all damn day. Normally I inhale a venti coffee on my way to work, but today I barely got through a couple of sips before tossing it. Something is definitely wrong. But I took a preggo test the nanosecond I got home tonight, and it came out negative. Whew. But what could it be? Doesn't feel like food poisoning, and it's been several days.

Psyched about my tattoo on Sunday, but the nausea better be gone. Can't imagine sitting still for hours feeling this awful. I like my tattoo artist and I refuse to puke on him. Plus, you're not supposed to vomit on freshly tattooed skin.

Thursday, April 6, 2017

Panicking.

As I got into the shower this morning, I noticed my abdomen had swelled up to monstrous proportions. I look eight months pregnant, which is confusing because I've lost weight recently (eating mostly plant-based foods and giving up dairy). But if I've lost weight, why is my belly so ginormous? I'm worried. Could it be leprosy, scarlet fever, or chicken pox?

Damn you, WebMD.

Friday, April 7, 2017

I showed Jon (my darling boyfriend since 2004) my stomach, and he looked alarmed and agreed something must be wrong. He made chicken noodle soup for dinner, but it tasted like dirt to me. He swore it tasted fine. This is scary—my taste buds are now malfunctioning. We're going to the emergency room tomorrow.

Saturday, April 8, 2017

Checked into the Cedars Sinai ER around eleven a.m. this morning.

Didn't have to wait long before I was in a comfy bed watching infomercials. Cheery nurses filed in and out. I had blood work, an ultrasound, and a CT scan. The doctor said it seemed like I'd passed a gallbladder stone. After several hours, one of my nurses came in and said I had to stay overnight. They wanted me to go upstairs for admitting and put on a gown.

But why? We were still waiting for my CT results, and I didn't have confirmation that a gallbladder stone was the demon inside me. She said she didn't have any information, other than a doctor's order to get me upstairs.

Well, this is slightly terrifying.

After they signed me in as a patient, I settled into my new room and sent Jon home to feed the cats. They hooked me up to an IV for fluids, and the machine screeched a horrendously loud alarm every time I bent my arm. Which made it impossible to sleep. Every time I drifted off, a *BEEP BEEP BEEP BEEP* jolted me awake. I could only nap in twenty-minute intervals. And I *still* didn't know why I had to stay overnight. Total misery. I just wanted to go home and crawl into my own bed.

Obviously, I had to miss tomorrow's tattoo appointment. I begrudgingly texted Dave and apologized for bailing since I was in the hospital. He completely understood, but I still want my tattoo, dammit.

Sunday, April 9, 2017

At eight a.m., a woman in blue scrubs woke me up. Her dark hair was pulled into a tight ponytail and her features were mild and unassuming—like a human version of toast without butter. Gripping a clipboard. she quietly greeted me and delivered the worst fucking news of my entire life.

"We have the results of your CT scan, and it's cancer."

Sorry, WHAT?...

WHAT?...

Wasn't it a gallbladder problem?

The lady's face was arranged into an expression of sympathy, but I couldn't accept her compassion—I didn't need it. I had no idea what she was talking about. It didn't compute. I saw spots. Everything went white, and I saw black spots. The air was thick.

That can't be right.

She stared at me and continued, "I know this is a lot of tough news…" but I couldn't pay attention. I only saw her mouth move. This made absolutely no sense. I didn't know what to say and eventually she left, probably to go drop a bomb on another unsuspecting patient.

I called Jon in tears, and he started crying and said he'd be by my side in fifteen minutes. I called my parents, sobbing. Alone. Petrified. *How the fuck did this happen?* How could I get the best news of my life (my book agent) followed by the worst?

Would I have six months to live? Would I die before my fiftieth birthday? My fortieth? Jesus Christ, I'd never visited Hawaii, gone skydiving, or owned a rescue dog!

Mom and Dad said they would come to L.A. next weekend. Between crying and hiccupping, I said they didn't have to, but they insisted. Jon showed up and we sat together, scared and weeping.

The afternoon was a haze, but soon the clouds parted and a magical man walked in. He introduced himself as my new oncologist, Dr. Andrew Li. An ovarian cancer specialist. A strikingly handsome source of light in a dark moment.

Are we sure he's a doctor, not a body double from Grey's Anatomy?

Dr. Li's bedside manner was calm and confident. His voice washed over us like a soothing balm that we so desperately needed. He explained that yes, my CT scan did indicate I could have ovarian cancer, but he was suspicious because I'm young and healthy, and there's no history of cancer in my family, so it didn't make sense.

SEE, LADY WHO WOKE ME UP THIS MORNING, IT DOESN'T MAKE ANY SENSE.

Thankfully, the tumors had not spread to my lymph nodes, nor were they inside my organs. But those nasty little growths were on my ovaries, uterus, liver, spleen (that explains the nagging pains in my abdomen), and scattered throughout my belly wall.

Dr. Li said I would need to stay another night so we could do a biopsy, then we'd know for sure what we're dealing with. And no matter what we're facing, he will help me get through it. What a fucking relief. I knew at that moment that Dr. Li is a precious gem and I started thinking about what to get him for Christmas. A framed photo of my ovaries, perhaps?

Monday, April 10, 2017

Slept like garbage again. Nurses came in and out every couple of hours. I constantly set off the screechy IV alarm. I felt sick with nerves. And the worst part is I couldn't eat or drink anything after midnight because of the upcoming biopsy. I normally drink a few liters of water every day, so the fluid denial was a special form of torture. My biopsy was scheduled for eleven a.m. and I watched the morning hours slowly tick by like a prisoner awaiting his release. Eventually noon rolled around. Then one. Then two. Then someone told me my biopsy was pushed to five p.m. Ugh. My mouth felt like sandpaper. The water deprivation was almost shittier than finding out I had cancer.

The biopsy itself was simple and quick. A little numbing here, a few needles there, and we were finished. I finally got discharged around eight o'clock and Dr. Li told me to come back on Friday for my biopsy results. What a goddamn shit show.

It felt amazing to be home and smother my cats with love, but my mind raced.

Do I seriously have cancer? Am I dying? Is this my new reality? Is this how my life was supposed to turn out?

Tuesday, April 11, 2017

I keep vacillating between, *There's absolutely no way I have cancer* and, *Oh my God, I can't believe I have cancer.* Work today was surreal. There's a bandage on my stomach from the biopsy and it reminds me things might be very different very soon.

The weirdest part was telling everyone what's going on. I missed work yesterday so my coworkers knew something was up, but I couldn't bring myself to say "ovarian cancer." All I could muster was, "I'm hoping it's not the big, scary thing" and tossing in a weak smile. Sitting at my desk helped me cope. Gus and Amy and Jake were warm and sympathetic, and we even cracked a few jokes. But my knees wouldn't stop shaking and I couldn't eat anything and an omnipresent rope of fear wrapped itself around my neck.

These tumors better be benign.

Mom, Dad, Rob (my eldest brother), and Brian (my middle brother) are all coming out this week. Thank God for my family. I'm beyond lucky. And I'm touched they're dropping everything to be by my side. The Tronic clan is nothing if not there for one another.

Thursday, April 13, 2017

Yay! Mom, Dad, and Brian arrived today. (Rob flies in tomorrow.) Their hugs and smiles and support instantly lifted my battered spirit. Jon and I brought them to Sun Cafe for dinner, one of our favorite vegan spots. We talked about everything over shared appetizers, and I finally started to feel better. Mom was right. She kept saying no matter what happens tomorrow, we will deal with it together, and my doctor will stand with me. But terrifying thoughts swirled around my mind. *It can't be cancer. But if it is, did I do this to myself? Am I gonna die young? Will I live long enough to walk down the aisle? Did I do something to deserve this?*

Anxiety does *not* mix well with vegan curry.

_____

Friday, April 14, 2017

Armed with Jon and my family, I anxiously shuffled into Cedars Sinai for the big results meeting. Was there any chance I didn't have cancer? Could I have some strange new disease that could be cured with chocolate and bong hits? Unfortunately, no. The very handsome Rockstar Cancer Ninja Dr. Li came in and introduced himself to my family. He calmly sat down. I almost threw up. He softly revealed that the biopsy indicated Stage Three ovarian cancer.

OH GOD. OH FUCK.

I immediately broke down in tears. As did Mom, Dad, Brian, and Jon.

Dr. Li wore an expression of true empathy on his adorable face. He waited a minute as my family and I composed ourselves, then assured me I would absolutely beat this. I have age on my side. I'm active and healthy. My cancer will respond amazingly to chemotherapy, and I will be cancer-free after this is done.

AH SHIT. It hadn't really hit me I would need chemo. My hair will fall out. My teeth will turn yellow. I'll have purple bags under my eyes. I'll look frail and sad and old and haggard like the people you see on those crappy Lifetime movies.

Dr. Li recommended an aggressive treatment plan, with nine consecutive weeks of chemo, then surgery (farewell, ovaries and uterus and possibly spleen), then nine more consecutive weeks of chemo. *So, basically this year will be as pleasant as a sandpaper enema.* I don't want to be bald. I've been growing my hair for the last six years, and now that'll (literally) go down the drain.

And with no ovaries or uterus, it will be difficult to conceive a child. Well, impossible, actually. Huh. So having kids is officially off the table. I guess this is just another piece of shitty information to make peace with. I suppose I could adopt, but I heard it's super expensive.

Can I put a baby on my Visa Rewards card? I probably have enough points saved up.

The nurse practitioner, Corina, gave me about 10,000 pieces of paperwork on everything from the side effects of chemo (yikes) to info on their psychology services (maybe necessary) to a list of Los Angeles wig-makers (definitely necessary) to a marijuana prescription (fuck yeah).

After the meeting, we zipped back to the hotel to meet Rob. We ordered cocktails at the hotel bar, then ate dinner at Granville Cafe. Despite the gloom hanging over my head, I felt a sense of safety with my family, like their love shielded me from imminent danger. I ordered a scrumptious avocado chicken salad, but when the food arrived, I couldn't eat. It smelled delicious, but each bite tasted like dust. I just couldn't believe this. It was real now.

I have fucking cancer inside my body.

Saturday, April 15, 2017

I'm trying to accept this bizarre new existence, but I feel like I'm in *Back To The Future II*, when Michael J. Fox takes the time machine to a new version of 1985, where everything is wrong and messed up. Jon said he wouldn't book any gigs for the next few months (he's a very talented drummer and plays in like eight bands). He also arranged to take every Friday off from work so he could sit with me during chemo. That made me cry, which made him cry. I better stock up on Kleenex.

Mom said we should get wigs today. I'm always down for shopping, but I dreaded this. I looked at my list of wig-makers, and the

first couple were on sketchy streets and didn't have websites, so…
bye. Another place had a Beverly Hills address and said, "Specialty Custom Wigs For Cancer And Chemotherapy Patients. By Appointment Only." Yep, sounds good! I called the number, knowing
they wouldn't have an appointment today but figured I could book
a time for next week. A sweet woman answered the phone and said
she did indeed have an opening in a couple of hours.

I hadn't thought about the cost of a wig until we pulled up to her
building, a sleek tower with valet parking and marble floors. Eeek.
We were escorted upstairs and met Amy, the beautiful wig-mak-
er. Her place reeked of style and elegance, with stunningly realistic
hairpieces scattered throughout. My eyes landed on a long, chestnut
wig I knew I'd take home (I ultimately named all my wigs, and this
one, Brigitte, turned out to be my favorite).

Amy told us about the wigs and explained she had alopecia which
means she had no hair on her body (including eyebrows and eyelashes). Wow. Her hair looked so real and she was clearly an expert
at drawing in eyebrows. I was obviously in good hands.

I found another piece I adored—a shorter brunette wig (Vicka)
that looked superb on me. While Amy's stylist trimmed both of
my wigs into natural, beautiful creations, Mom tried on a couple
of pieces and bought one that transformed her into a Swedish rock
star. Dad and Rob sat in the living room with Amy, and I could hear
them getting along famously.

When my wigs were ready, I nearly had an aneurysm when Amy
said the total came to 11,000 bucks. Uh. That's practically half a year
of my college tuition. Thank God Dad felt awful about the cancer
thing, so he paid up with little complaining. And hey, you can't put
a price on feeling good, right?

After Amy's we meandered over to CityWalk, a touristy delight
for people who love chain restaurants, tacky souvenirs, and obnoxiously oversized neon signs. During dinner, my pulse felt fast and I

kept having heart palpitations. Dad timed my pulse several times, which made me even more nervous. He chalked it up to anxiety, but I swore I was having a heart attack.

Can cancer cause heart attacks?

———————

Sunday, April 16, 2017

Happy Easter, I guess. This morning I posted the "Facebook Cancer Announcement" to let my FB friends know what's going on. It was a long thoughtful post, and the responses blew me away. I got messages, comments, and emails from so many folks—close buddies, former work acquaintances, and people I hadn't seen since high school. A couple of girls from my hometown who themselves had beaten cancer sent me heartfelt, comforting messages. One gal told me, "The main thing you need is strength. And from what I remember about you, you've got no shortage. Your spunky attitude and sense of humor are gonna help kick this thing in the ass. Cancer doesn't stand a chance!"

Girl, my spunky attitude and sense of humor are hiding under an avalanche of terror.

Rob needed to run a few errands, so I brought the gang to a nearby shopping plaza. As we pulled up, Jon noticed a wig shop next to Whole Foods. Oooh! I popped in and scanned the rows of hair. The wigs weren't as nice as Amy's, but they weren't as expensive, either. I tried on a couple of options and walked out with a chocolate brown piece (Mandy), a slutty-looking layered piece with terrible orange highlights (TammiLynn), and a fire-engine red bob (Alexis). My wig collection is really picking up some steam.

For my family's final day in L.A. I brought them to another vegan hotspot, Gracias Madre. We had dinner on the beautiful patio, and it was the perfect way to cap off their trip. My parents kept saying how good they felt about everything after meeting Dr. Li. They'd previously wanted me to get a second opinion in Boston, but once they met my Rockstar Cancer Ninja, they knew I wouldn't get better care anywhere else. Their confidence gave me confidence. *Maybe I'll make it out alive after all.*

Monday, April 17, 2017

Back at work after the big news. It's so bizarre telling everyone, "Yes, I have cancer." It still doesn't fit right, kinda like those jeans you used to wear before you put on ten pounds. *This isn't me. I'm healthy. I'm loud and sarcastic. I'm hyper and I talk too fast. I'm not a cancer patient. Except I suppose I am.*

My coworkers reacted the exact way I imagine I would if the situation were reversed:

1) Widen eyeballs
2) Tip head back slightly
3) Wince and shake head
4) Say something encouraging
5) Offer hug
6) Say something lighthearted and possibly make tiny joke

During the rush-hour commute home, I concluded there are three things I'm most dreading: my first chemo session, shaving my head, and surgery. My debut chemo session is this Friday, so there's not a lot of time to sit around and freak out. Is it gonna hurt? Make me puke on the spot? I envision myself on the couch with my head in a bucket for the next six months. I hope I don't miss a lot of work. God, cancer is so *inconvenient.*

Wednesday, April 19, 2017

Today I lost my Pot Shop virginity. Many of my California friends consider the dispensaries a second home, but this was a new experience for me. I was overwhelmed by all the shelves of nuggets, edibles, and oils. I didn't know where to start. The guy behind the counter told me to take a mix of the CBD and THC oil to help reduce the tumors and improve any appetite/nausea issues. Cool! I grabbed a bunch of edibles and the dude threw in a few extra cookies for free. I think I like this place.

My brother Brian, who's into the yoga/alternative healing scene, wants me to start meditating. He said it'll reduce my anxiety, mellow my stress levels, and improve my self-awareness. I'm intrigued, but usually I get those same benefits from alcohol and carbs. Brian's sweet girlfriend, Anita, emailed me several guided mediations so I could test the waters. I haven't met her in person yet (they live in Washington D.C.), but I was touched she took the time to send me some digital restoration.

Brian also suggested I see this legendary energy healer in Los Angeles named Mahankirn. Brian said she's the granddaughter of a famous Yogi Master who trained her in Sat Nam Rasayan (the sacred art of healing with inner silence). She offers a healing treatment called Bound Lotus, a practice that allegedly clears out your negative energy and resets your nervous system. Brian said I don't have to do anything during the session, just lie there and relax.

Great. With a treacherous road ahead, I'm down for anything that will help me relax. *But really, is it even possible to relax when you have hostile little cancer cells feeding on your insides?*

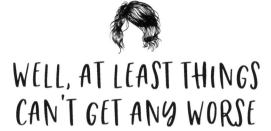

PART TWO

WELL, AT LEAST THINGS CAN'T GET ANY WORSE

Friday, April 21, 2017

Well, here we go. Chemo Session #1.

Slept terribly. Nervous as hell. I had a feeling it would be a long day because I would get two drugs administered, Taxol and Carboplatin. Every Friday for nine weeks I'd get Taxol, and every third Friday would be a Double-Dipper day with *both* Taxol and Carboplatin. I guess the combination of drugs is more effective for treating ovarian cancer than just one drug.

Last week, Rockstar Cancer Ninja Dr. Li gave me an overview about chemo, but uncertainty and fear radiated throughout my insides. Would it hurt? Would I barf all over my sweatpants? Would my head spin around like the girl in *The Exorcist*? I probably should have asked these questions earlier, but they didn't occur to me until the concept of chemo became a reality—i.e., when shit got real.

I didn't know what to bring, so I stuffed my bags with pj's, a couple of comedy memoirs (figured I could use some laughs), pillows, blankets, snacks, drinks, an iPad, phone chargers, sandwiches, water, more water, extra socks, and lotion.

Jon and I checked in to Cedars at nine a.m. and were escorted to the Procedures Center. Before starting chemo, I needed a "passport" installed in my upper arm. Since I'm having chemo every Friday for nine consecutive weeks, it would be too hard on my veins to poke a fresh line each session, so they put this weird thing under my bicep skin that stays attached to my veins. Then they just poke a teeny hole in my arm and attach my chemo IV to the passport every week. I didn't even know this existed. Thanks, advances in medical technology!

We chilled in the waiting room for a while. Then an hour passed. Then another. They were running behind, and the anxiety ate at my stomach like a piranha. Finally, after nearly three hours, I changed into a gown and they numbed my arm. While I lay on the table waiting for the doctor, the techs and nurses chatted about their lunches and weekend plans. One of the techs had messed up his ankle playing basketball, and the pretty nurse loved her kale salad from the cafe across the street.

How fucking weird. They're here for just another day of work, casually discussing food and sports, while I'm nestled under layers of sterile surgical blankets with a mask and numb arm, wondering what the fuck I'm doing here. How I got cancer. How I lost the shittiest lottery on earth. Wondering if I will survive.

Finally the doctor came in and took about forty-five minutes to get the passport set up. Afterwards I got dressed and we went back downstairs for blood work and to meet Dr. Li before kicking off my first chemo treatment.

His reassuring face calmed me down. This meeting was a lot more relaxed and positive compared to the last time we saw him. I asked a billion questions about side effects and hair loss and diet, and Dr. Li patiently explained everything. Before each chemo session, they would test my blood to make sure my body could handle the onslaught of poison coming its way. Once my blood gets processed in the lab (which should take around forty-five minutes), and I get clearance to proceed, the nurses administer my pre-meds (steroids,

Ativan, fluids, anti-allergy and anti-nausea medications). After the pre-meds, I start the actual chemo infusion—which means just sitting on the bed until the whole bag of toxic liquid seeps through my IV. Easy peasy.

Every three weeks, we'd test my CA-125 (which indicates the level of tumor protein in my cells—the lower the number, the better) to keep tabs on my progress. Dr. Li gave me a few final words of encouragement, then it was party time.

A nurse brought me and Jon to a private little room with a flat screen TV and its own bathroom. I settled onto the cozy bed and found some good infomercials to watch. (Don't judge me, but I'm obsessed with the Copper Chef cooking infomercials. The cheesy, saccharine-sweet energy oozing from the over-enthusiastic host makes me happy. Plus, I enjoy looking at unhealthy food.)

My nurse began the pre-meds, and as they kicked in, a kind gal named Daniella talked to me about genetics. We went through my family history, and she explained that I had to be tested for the BRCA gene mutation, which predisposes women to breast and ovarian cancer. By then, the Ativan was meandering through my system. I was super woozy and I just kept nodding so we could finish and I could lie down. (Note to Cedars: maybe think about sending in the geneticist *before* administering the snoozy stuff?)

Wooooo. Once the Ativan *really* kicked in, everything became floaty and OK. Chemo is OK. This bed is OK. Cancer is OK...And this turkey sandwich is fucking *delicious*! I love Ativan. This is fun!

We went home after three short hours, armed with Compazine (for nausea); Zofran (also for nausea, but stronger than Compazine—but insurance won't cover as much so use sparingly); Temazepam (for insomnia); and Colace and MiraLax (to...uh...help move things along—apparently the anti-nausea meds can be *very* constipating). I felt sleepy and kind of hopeful. That wasn't so bad. If every week is this easy, I've totally got this.

Saturday, April 22, 2017

A little queasy today, but I took a Compazine and it cleared up. Wanted to go out for dinner, so Jon took me to Musso & Frank's. We typically save that for special occasions, but I deserved a special treat. I ate a CBD gummy as we left the house because I knew I shouldn't have a cocktail. I'm *allowed* to have alcohol, but since your liver is the organ that processes both chemo and booze, you shouldn't add additional stress to it.

I enjoyed venturing out, doing something normal, and eating an exquisite meal. I didn't feel stoned from the gummy, just relaxed and chill. During dinner, I kept looking around at other people engrossed in conversation. I felt a stab of envy that they could eat their chicken and steaks and not worry about evil tumors inside their bodies. Lucky fuckers. Do they even know how good they have it not bearing this burden? Would I ever be like them again, able to worry about normal shit? Then I realized I have no idea if they're going through tough times. They could be here, enjoying their food, but reeling from a divorce. Or death in the family. Or trying not to fart in front of their date.

Monday, April 24, 2017

Oh God. So this is the nausea I'd been warned about.

Woke up dry heaving at five a.m. Took a Compazine and went back to sleep. Woke up queasy two hours later. Took a Zofran. Started to feel better and hopped in the shower. As I dried off, a major case of the dry heaves came back. *Fuck. Can I even make it to work today?* Took a quick ten-minute nap (still wearing a towel) and forced down some cucumber slices and water. Felt better so I went to work.

Everyone was supportive and asked about chemo. During a

meeting, I sat next to Jeff, the CEO, and he'd just poured a fresh cup of French vanilla coffee. The repulsive smell coated my nose and I almost threw up on the table.

I'm digging the meditations that Anita (my brother's girlfriend) sent me. My goal is to meditate every day. I enjoy listening to the lady's soft, soothing voice after I crawl into bed. I'll throw in my earbuds and try to lose myself in the chill background organ music. It almost seems like the Universe is whispering to me, "Shhh…you'll be OK." Most nights I fall asleep before the end of the meditation and I'll wake up in the middle of the night with the headphones pressing into my cheek.

Tuesday, April 25, 2017

I keep forgetting I have cancer. I'm glad the initial chemo is over, but the next scary milestone is Sunday—my big head shave. I'm gonna miss my hair. I've been savoring the sensation every time I brush it, wash it, and run my fingers through the long silky strands. I even like pulling my hair and feeling the tug on my scalp. Soon I won't have any of these luxuries. I guess baldness will become another "new normal."

Had another violent case of the dry heaves this morning while I brushed my teeth. It was brutal. I think the anti-nausea meds aren't working as well as they're supposed to. The dry heaving came on suddenly but passed after a few minutes. The upside is I've lost about fifteen pounds. *What an effortless diet!*

Despite the omnipresent queasiness, I love being at work. We're super busy, and I'm grateful to have positive things to focus on. Keeping my mind occupied can help stave off the nausea. And with the cancer quips flying around, it's impossible not to giggle. It may seem weird to joke about cancer, but making light of the situation makes it less scary. Gus, one of my coworkers, asked me to email him a file, and I told him no, because cancer patients shouldn't have to work. We laughed and it felt good.

Wednesday, April 26, 2017

Today I visited Mahankirn, the magical energy healer my brother recommended. She lives a beautiful house filled with colors, cozy furniture, and peaceful vibes. I felt comfortable around her right away. Her piercing blue eyes and inviting smile melted away my uncertainty about the session. We introduced ourselves and settled onto a shaggy rug. I told her about my diagnosis, and she assured me she's worked with a lot of cancer survivors.

She explained that our mental health is vital to our physical health. She made an interesting point about my anxiety (that butterfly/rollercoaster sensation in my stomach) being in the same location as my tumors.

Huh. Maybe she's on to something.

Today we would do a healing treatment called Bound Lotus, which has roots in Kundalini, Ashtanga, and Hatha Yoga. (Don't ask me what that means—I later looked up some info online, and it said, "Bound Lotus allows you to merge into the spirit realm where all healing is possible, providing many physical, mental, emotional and spiritual benefits.") We'd start with vibrations to clear away my negative energy, then begin the treatment, where she remains in a very uncomfortable-looking position for thirty minutes, while I sit still and breathe. OK, sounds easy enough.

Mahankirn told me to lie down and placed several bowls on my body. I was kinda hoping she'd fill them with popcorn, but instead she gently tapped each one, and vibrations soared throughout my insides. It was an odd sensation, but a soothing one. This went on for about fifteen minutes, and my mind seemed a lot less chatty than normal. I then sat Indian-style against a wall, while Mahankirn arranged her body in a pose I'd never be able to do—sitting Indian-style while leaning forward all the way to the ground. My back hurt just looking at her. She had music playing quietly in the background, and I almost fell asleep. As my level of awareness softened, my fears and stresses drifted away. *I'm gonna be OK. I'm gonna get through this. I'm gonna fix everything that's wrong and live a long happy life. But damn, I could really go for some popcorn.*

When we finished, I opened my eyes and emerged back into reality, shocked at how good I felt. My head was clear. My shoulders and limbs felt warm and loose. The tension, both mentally and physically, had completely dissipated. I felt light, as if the Universe hugged me. Hmm…perhaps I'd been too quick to judge Eastern medicine all my life. I asked if we could do another Bound Lotus healing, and she said no, this was a one-time treatment, but we could do a different healing called Sat Nam Rasayan. Great! I didn't know what that entailed, but maybe the silver lining of my cancer situation was to open me up to new spiritual experiences.

Friday, April 28, 2017

Chemo Session #2!

I only had Taxol today, so it was a short afternoon. (The Double-Dipper days—Taxol plus Carboplatin—take much longer because I receive double the amount of chemo.) Gobbled up another heavenly turkey sandwich and it was just as tasty as last week. I also snacked on dozens of Honey Graham Crackers that Jon retrieved from the goody bowls at the nurse's station.

Chemo isn't that terrible. Once that amazing Ativan hits your system, you barely even notice you're getting pumped full of poison. (OK, fine, technically it's not poison, since chemo doesn't kill you—but it does destroy your healthy cells along with cancer cells. And because of the brutal side effects, it seems like you're getting sicker even though you're actually getting better.) Plus, you have lots of time to watch TV, so Jon and I binge-watched *Nurse Jackie* on his iPad. Great show—solid writing, quality acting, and I love the way you can't decide if the main character is a sinner or a saint.

During treatment, the Cedars nutritionist visited my bay and we talked about my diet. Her name is L.J. and she's from Connecticut. I liked her right away. I told her about my current diet, and she said to keep doing what I'm doing (minimize the sugar, alcohol, and processed stuff, and pack in tons of fruits, veggies, and lean proteins). L.J. acknowledged when you're feeling awful from chemo, it's difficult to adhere to a perfectly healthy diet, because you need to eat anything that doesn't gross you out (which will be everything). She mentioned my taste buds will probably change, and I may end up hating foods I once loved (and vice versa).

Rockstar Cancer Ninja Dr. Li said my hair would start falling out between Sessions #3 and #4, and it's common to wake up with chunks of hair on your pillow. But I can't bear to watch even one strand fall out. My self-esteem and feminine essence are synonymous with my long hair. Seeing a pile of limp strands in my bed will break me. So I'm gonna gather all my courage and have my stylist, Matthew, shave my head this weekend. I could probably do it at home, but I think I'd suffer an emotional meltdown. And cleaning up the mess would be annoying. Matthew always blasts upbeat music when I get my hair done, so I know he'll turn this into something fun instead of something sad. Bald is beautiful, right? Jon is a peach and said he'd shave his head too.

Sunday, April 30, 2017

BALD. I'M SO FUCKING BALD NOW.

I knew this day was coming, but it didn't prepare me for the reality of having *no* hair. Jon volunteered to go first and Matthew threw on some Madonna. I pretended to be calm, but my stomach was in knots. My hair is part of my identity. Will I even feel feminine anymore? I tried to remain brave as Jon's blondish spikes flittered off. He looked sexy with his cropped 'do, but I dreaded my moment in the chair.

I sat down and braced myself. The buzz from the razor grated my nerves, like when you're at the dentist and the loud *ZZZZZZ* assaults your brain. Matthew went to work on the first strands and I helplessly watched as my gorgeous locks fell lifelessly to the ground.

As more of my scalp emerged, I realized I didn't look so awful. Thankfully I don't have a lumpy head. I'd kinda been afraid of looking like Dan Aykroyd in *Coneheads* (or Sloth from *The Goonies*). Maybe I'll eventually embrace this haircut but I dislike how masculine it makes me feel. Fuck, I should go buy a dress or bake a cake or something.

––––––––––

Monday, May 1, 2017

My boss Jeff completely surprised me today. He pulled me aside for a meeting and I immediately tensed up and wondered if I was about to get the, *We-know-you're-going-through-a-lot-right now-so-maybe-we-should-cut-you-down-to-part-time-or-better-yet-maybe-you-should-take-some-time-off-and-quit* speech.

But, no. Jeff kindly explained he knew firsthand how tough health problems can be.

"Seriously," he said. "I get what it's like. I had to take two months off from a prior job to recover from surgery. And my boss didn't give me the support that I needed. So I want to be there for you. The whole team is here for you."

I exhaled a breath I didn't even realize I'd been holding.

"For real. If you need Fridays off for chemo, that's totally cool. If you don't feel good on the days surrounding your treatment, you can just work from home. The most important thing is your health. We need you to be healthy and strong so you can keep kicking ass here."

I nodded my head through a stream of tears. *How fucking lucky am I?!*

Tuesday, May 2, 2017

Today at work we met with one of our new clients. She's completely flawless—shiny hair, smooth skin, impeccable makeup, expensive clothes. She exudes glamour and elegance. During the meeting, I wondered if she could tell I was wearing a wig. Could she sense my baldness like a magical glitzy bloodhound? I didn't bother to put on makeup so my frumpiness had truly reached Level-Ten-Hag.

Jeff brought in a huge cup of coffee and the aroma immediately activated my upchuck reflex. I ran to the bathroom and splashed water on my face. After a few deep breaths, I snuck to the kitchen and forced down a couple of snacks. I remember Dr. Li saying that eating throughout the day can help minimize nausea, but it's hard to shove food down your throat when you're certain it'll come back up. And I'm saddened by how much coffee grosses me out. Don't worry Starbucks—one day you and I will reunite.

Friday, May 5, 2017

Chemo Session #3! This marks the end of Cycle #1, which means just five cycles left (one cycle is three weeks). Today I had a super hot male nurse with a wicked good sense of humor. He kept saying that Jon was stealing food from dying patients as Jon snacked on crackers from the nurse's station.

Turkey sandwiches are my official ritual now. I actually look forward to those. A true delicacy in the chemo ward.

I wore my TammiLynn wig during the session, and her bad '90s-era dye job (think: chunky, unblended highlights that look like giant stripes across your head) matched the wood panels in the chemo bay. I had one of those "Who Wore It Better" moments between my wig and the wall. I think my wig pulled it off better. Thankfully my blood levels are decent, and we're one week closer to getting this shit done.

––––––––––

Monday, May 8, 2017

Felt good today. Seems like the post-Taxol weeks are less riddled with sickness than the Double-Dipper weeks.

Jake (the awesome exec who hired me) has been on vacation and he'll return to the office on Wednesday. I'm excited about working on our new marketing campaigns. There's huge potential for them to succeed.

I've also been thinking about traveling. Jake went to Iceland for his trip, and a few of my friends make a point to travel at least once a year. I should do that. I've been to the Dominican Republic and Jamaica for family vacations (those were spectacular), but I've always wanted to check out Greece, Croatia, Tuscany, and Australia. Maybe I can start putting a few bucks away from each paycheck. Cancer has shown me that you can't wait to make shit happen—you gotta do it now.

––––––––––

Wednesday, May 10, 2017

God hates me.

I lost my job today.

Completely unexpected. When I got back from lunch, Jeff wanted to chat. The moment I sat down, I knew I was a goner. I could tell Jeff felt bad. His cheeks were flushed and he spoke rapidly.

"Kim, I know the timing is terrible, but I'll be honest: we're in a horrible financial crisis. Our next round of investor funds is taking way longer than we thought it would, and two new clients are dragging their feet in signing a contract and therefore we don't have their deposits…"

I leaned back in my chair, hoping I could sink into the floor.

"This is purely a financial decision. If things don't change, we won't last more than a couple of months. But we truly appreciate everything you've done for us. We hate that things turned out this way and we wanna make sure you know you did a great job…"

Blah blah blah. Fuck.

I know he's telling the truth, but this stings. Work was my escape. My safe haven. What the hell am I going to do with my free time now? I'll definitely work on writing my book, but what about money? No one is going to hire me. Picture this:

Interviewer: Well, Kim, we're very impressed with your work experience and portfolio, and we'd like to offer you the position.

Me: Thank you! I'm so excited and I truly appreciate the opportunity!

Interviewer: Great! When can you start?

Me: Well, here's the thing…I have cancer and I'm undergoing chemotherapy, so I'll need every Friday off until September. Is that cool? Oh, and I'm having surgery at the end of June, so I'll need a few weeks off to recover from that. And I tend to feel like shit on Mondays because of the chemo, so I just want to make sure there's a bathroom near my desk.

Interviewer: It was nice meeting you, but the position is no longer available.

Me: OK, can you at least validate my parking?

Interviewer: No.

Friday, May 12, 2017

Chemo Session #4! Today is a Double-Dipper Taxol and Carboplatin day so I'll feel crappy next week. (I've noticed that I usually feel OK the day or two after chemo because the pre-meds are still in my system; it's four or five days *after* treatment that the queasiness rears its monstrous head.) But we got some great news. My tumor marker (the CA-125) was 157 today, and when we began it was 380. My tumors are shrinking, which means treatment is effective.

I may have no job, but at least chemo is working. Zing.

My weight continues to plummet—I'm down to 162 now (I was about 170 when we started). I love it because my skinny jeans will soon fit, but hate it because my beloved boobs are getting smaller. I already had to give up my hair, but my boobs are my prized possession. Time to invest in some cushy push-up bras from Victoria's Secret. Maybe Dad won't mind buying me those. I mean, he already threw down eleven grand on hair, so what's a few hundo on some over-the-shoulder-boulder-holders? I feel guilty he's dropped so much dough on my vanity, but thankfully he made the wise career choice to be a doctor, and it affords him the privilege of pissing away his hard-earned money on my stupid bullshit.

After chemo, Jon and I went to our buddy Courtney's house for a BBQ. I am obsessed with her pit bull, Tank, so I spent most of the evening spooning him on the kitchen floor. The rest of the time I caught up with gals I hadn't seen since my diagnosis. I loved being around such lovely people and they fawned over my hair (I wore Brigitte because she's the silkiest and most luxurious of my hairpieces), and I finally felt good about myself. Actually, I felt so good that I let the girls see my bald head. It was a bit raw and scary, but I knew no one judged me, and I felt safe enough to let them see the real me. But seriously, fuck baldness.

Also, I ate pork for the first time in over a decade. Before this ordeal, I'd been eating mostly plant-based because I feel bad about eating animals. I mean, I'm crazy about cats and dogs, so how is slaughtering a farm animal any different? But I just started craving chicken so I'm trying to listen to my body. Tonight, my body said it wanted the scrumptious pulled pork that taunted me from those foil trays on Courtney's table.

#SorryPiggies #JustATemporaryCarnivore

Sunday, May 14, 2017

Hi, my name is Kim, and I'm addicted to wigs.

I wanted more colors, so I visited the same shop where I bought Mandy, TammiLynn, and Alexis. I tried on a few pieces and walked out with a neon blue bob (Smurfette) and a wavy hot pink number (Lacy). If nothing else, I'm gathering inspiration for what I'll do once my hair grows back.

After shopping, I saw Mahankirn (the energy healer who did my Bound Lotus treatment last month) for our first Sat Nam Rasayan session. A quick Google search told me that the process involves "... holding a neutral, contemplative state of awareness, being aware of everything—all sensations—then allowing the resistances to change as you hold your state of awareness." *Huh?*

I got to her house, and we had a quick chat. I told her how much I loved the Bound Lotus treatment, but I'm having a tough time staying in a positive mindset—like, is that even possible when you're fighting cancer?

"Yes. Of course. Remember, cancer isn't what defines you. It's something that's happening TO you, but it isn't WHO YOU ARE."

I liked that distinction. We began the healing session, and I repeated the sentiment in my head. As I lay on her comfy blanket, and she gently placed her hands on my arms, shoulders, stomach, and thighs, I thought about what she said. If this is only something that's happening TO me, it doesn't have power to dictate my life. I can still be the upbeat, annoying, foul-mouthed, loudmouth maniac that I am...not a weak cancer patient.

After thirty minutes, she told me to open my eyes, and everything felt right with the world. I don't really understand the science or spirituality behind Sat Nam Rasayan, but I felt happily mushy, like I'd taken three Vicodin.

Spiritual Vicodin. That'd make a great band name.

————

Monday, May 15, 2017

Total. Emotional. Fucking. Meltdown.

I was in the bathroom putting on my face lotion when I noticed something disturbing. As I gently smeared the cream across my cheeks, I suddenly saw rows of white hair standing up like little soldiers.

WHAT IS THIS?! Peach fuzz. On my cheeks and around my sideburns area. I freaked out and started bawling hysterically. As if I didn't feel ugly enough, with my bald head and shrinking breasts, now I was growing a *PEACH BEARD?!*

Jon rushed in and tried to calm me down. He grabbed the clippers and helped me shave the fuzz off, but I cried so hard I couldn't stay still. This was by far the most humiliating thing I'd ever experienced, much worse than the head shave. Part of the shock stemmed from the fact that I'd had no warning. Rockstar Cancer Ninja Dr. Li *definitely* didn't mention a lady beard as a chemo side effect.

After Jon left for work, I continued sobbing. My womanhood seemed to be slipping away. No hair. Smaller boobs. Soon I wouldn't have ovaries or a uterus. What was left?

I knew cancer would suck, but I hadn't anticipated a total robbery of my femininity.

I wiped away the snot and tears and scoured online cancer forums for answers. Turns out, many women experienced the same hair growth, and it wasn't permanent. I took a little comfort in knowing the hair would fall out, but the trauma of seeing that fuzz in my reflection completely fucked me up. Would Jon even be able to look at me in the same way now? I'm all for doing things together with your boyfriend, but shaving my face was not a team-building exercise I ever care to repeat.

Tuesday, May 16, 2017

This morning Daniella, the Cedars geneticist, called with my results: I tested positive for the BRCA1 gene mutation.

The BRCA gene makes you high-risk for developing breast and ovarian cancer. But since I already have ovarian cancer, does this mean I'm in the clear moving forward, or do I have a high risk of getting breast cancer after this? I'll need to ask Dr. Li, because I can't imagine the pain of going through this again. I was so upset I didn't think to ask Daniella while we were on the phone.

Another. Total. Emotional. Meltdown. (A few rounds of sobbing, hiccupping, gasping for air, breaking a plate, then more sobbing.)

The gene mutation comes from Dad's side. Thanks a lot, Dad! He was devastated when I told him, as if he personally gave me cancer. I said to calm down, 'cuz really, it's not his fault. No one on his side ever got tested. But now that he feels bad, maybe he'll be willing to buy me those expensive bras...

Thursday, May 18, 2017

Now that I have the BRCA results, I've been thinking about kids a lot. Obviously I won't be able to have them, but even if I could, would I want to, knowing this gene mutation would predispose them to cancer? Maybe not. I think I'm coming to terms with adoption. Funny how I never really wanted kids before, but now that the option is taken away, it's difficult to accept.

Jon had a rough day. I think the pressure of taking care of me, coupled with the stress of the situation, had built and built and built until finally he exploded. He went to a bar after work, and I could see he was drunk, but more significantly, something inside of him was broken. He was in a dark headspace, exactly where I'd been earlier in the week.

Through fits of tears, he confessed he was scared about my upcoming surgery and felt horrible I might be at the hospital alone while he was at work. He'd been shattered to see me so depressed a few days ago (*fuck off, peach beard*) and feared I would break down like that every week. I tried to assure him everything would be OK. I told him we have good days and bad days, and we're just doing our best to get through this. But nothing I said helped.

Honestly, I knew this would happen at some point. I've been meditating, and I dragged him to a yoga class, but I didn't see him making an effort to take care of himself mentally or emotionally. Poor guy just needed a release. I'm hoping he can get to a better headspace, because he deserves to be happy and fulfilled, and this is just as challenging for him as it is for me. Actually, this is probably worse for him, because he's sort of a helpless bystander.

Friday, May 19, 2017

Chemo Session #5 knocked out! Boom.

Super psyched we've only got a few more treatments before surgery. Up until now, my blood levels had been decent, but today my nurse said my hemoglobin levels were too low, and I'd need a transfusion after the chemo. Not a huge deal, but the transfusion tacked on two extra hours, and we ended up being at Cedars for seven hours. My back was killing me, and I wanted to suggest they invest in those $3,000 massage chairs from Brookstone.

I wore my bright blue wig (Smurfette) to chemo, and a few other patients came by to compliment me. I'm glad I could provide a moment of brightness in their day. I'm also down to 155 pounds now, which is pleasing to see on the scale. Cancer is seriously the easiest diet I've ever been on. I haven't weighed this little since 2003. My poor boobs. If they don't bounce back to their original fullness, I'll need to consider silicone implants.

Sunday, May 21, 2017

Woke up thinking about my job situation (well, lack thereof). Since surgery is just around the corner, it doesn't make sense to look for a new full-time gig. I'd been so happy to ditch the freelance life a few months ago, but it looks like I'll have to return with my tail between my legs.

Went to a patio party this afternoon. My buddy Heather (who owns a superb vegan cookie company) was selling her vegan ice cream sandwiches, and there was music, bingo, and vegan tacos. For the most part, I've been eating clean and avoiding sugar since the diagnosis. But today I lost my resolve and packed in a few tacos and two ice cream sandwiches. Fuck it, I'm only human. I enjoyed every bite.

Jon won the first round of bingo, and it was a great way to end the week. We're both in much better spirits, and I'm happy we can still have wonderful days.

Monday, May 22, 2017

Mom and Dad are debating whether they want to be here for my actual surgery, or wait until I'm healed and healthy enough to skip around town. I think it makes more sense to wait until I'm healed. If they come out while I'm in the hospital, we'll barely get to spend any time together, and I'll be drugged up on my bed (fun for me but not for them).

I was exhausted today. Took three naps throughout the afternoon, which is way out of character for me. I did manage a trip to the gym, but my body is weak. I used to run for miles, and now I'm wiped out from a gentle twenty minutes on the elliptical. I know I'll get strong again, but it's depressing to see how much I've regressed. I can't have saggy boobs *and* a saggy ass.

Funny how I never appreciated the privileges of exercising or having children until they were taken away.

_____

Tuesday, May 23, 2017

My poor scalp is getting super patchy, so I wear bandanas around the house and avoid mirrors. At least my teeth aren't yellow, and I don't have purple bags under my eyes—yet. And that hideous peach fuzz has barely grown back, so no meltdowns for now.

Psyched that Friday marks the end of Chemo Cycle #2. Then just a few more sessions and it's surgery time. I think I want a farewell party for my ovaries and uterus. Seriously. I want a uterus-shaped cake. Wouldn't that be fun?

I started taking CBD oil at night, and it soothes my anxiety. Glad I live in California and can easily obtain this wondrous extract. Prior to my cancer shit storm, I didn't know anything about CBD. According to Leafly.com, "Cannabidiol (CBD) is one of many cannabinoid molecules produced by cannabis, second only to THC in abundance...While THC is the principal psychoactive component of cannabis and has certain medical uses, CBD stands out because it is both non-intoxicating and displays a broad range of potential medical applications. These properties make it especially attractive as a therapeutic agent." So basically, CBD doesn't get you high but delivers all the mental and physical benefits from the cannabis plant, like reducing anxiety, reducing pain, and helping you sleep.

Teenage me would be proud of all the cannabis products currently stocked in my cabinets.

Thursday, May 25, 2017

Went for an amazing run yesterday. Sprinted up a hill and realized maybe I'm not as weak as I thought. Today's workout was solid as well. Maybe I'm getting my stride back, both literally and figuratively.

Tonight Jon and I went to a birthday party at a Tex-Mex restaurant. The margaritas were huge, and it was hard to sit there and not order a cocktail, but I resisted. However, I did indulge in five pounds of chips and salsa, and my stomach got angry about it. Oh, and I inhaled a red velvet cupcake, so I gotta be more on point with my eating habits. Tumors love sugar, and I want those suckers to shrivel up and die.

I definitely want a hysterectomy party. I'm envisioning a giant realistic uterus cake and sweet little ovary cupcakes on the side. I've had my ovaries and uterus for thirty-six years, and they deserve a proper send off. Maybe I'll do balloons and karaoke with a solid rendition of "I Will Remember You" by Sarah McLachlan.

I finally emailed Jill (my literary agent) an initial draft of my manuscript. I've been working on this collection of essays for over three years and this is my baby (which is great, considering I won't be able to actually have a baby). I'm nervous and excited to get her feedback.

Best case scenario: "Kim, I love it, and you're the best writer in the world, and I can easily get this published."

Worst case scenario: "Kim, my five-year-old nephew can write better than this. You have no idea how to tell a story, and you should just stick to writing poetry on bathroom walls with a Sharpie."

Friday, May 26, 2017

Today was the epitome of a yin and yang day. It was supposed to be Chemo Session #6 (marking the end of Cycle #2), but after the nurse got my blood results, she said we couldn't proceed because my white blood cells were too low. So now everything is delayed a week, including surgery. Sucks.

Jon and I met with Daniella, the Cedars geneticist. I was hoping since I have cancer now, I'd be free and clear from it in the future, like this was my Cancer Hallway Pass and I'd never get a recurrence or develop breast cancer. Sadly, this is not the case.

Daniella said my chances of getting breast cancer are really high, between fifty and eighty-five percent.

OH GOD. OH FUCK.

More shitty news. How much more can I take?

I immediately decided to get a double mastectomy and breast implants. (Weird that I'd thought about implants a couple of weeks ago anyway.) I can't live the rest of my life fearing those horrible words again, "You have cancer." No. Better to nip this in the proverbial bud and get fake boobs. It's kind of a no-brainer: perky breasts, peace of mind, and insurance will cover everything. *Maybe it's not so bad.*

I also discovered that my post-surgery chemo sessions will be different since I'm BRCA-positive. Instead of these easy-peasy IV chemo treatments in my arm once a week, we'll need to install a passport in my belly and administer the drugs through my arm *and* tummy. One day will be the IV arm treatment, the next day will be the passport belly treatment, then the following three days I'll come back to the hospital for IV fluids to flush my kidneys. The following week will be just the IV arm treatment, and the next week will be off, then that cycle is repeated two more times.

Sigh. Any other ways you'd like to shit on me, Universe? Maybe a flat tire on the way home? Flood in my apartment?

I said it before, and I'll say it again ... cancer is so fucking *inconvenient.*

But the day took a positive turn when, out of nowhere, my brother Brian and his girlfriend Anita showed up at my chemo bay. They live in D.C., so it blew my mind to see them casually stroll up. I cried like an infant. Turns out they're in town for a wedding, and they wanted to surprise me.

They came back to my place to hang for a bit. After all the harsh news recently, their uplifting spirits eased my inner turmoil. We had dinner at The Spot, L.A.'s oldest vegetarian restaurant. The food was delectable and the conversation was exactly what I needed—laughter, love, and empathy. Tomorrow they're going to a wedding but we'll hang out on Sunday. I wanna take them to Gracias Madre, the vegan Mexican place I took my family last month.

Yep, nothing is better than family. *Viva La Tronics!*

Saturday, May 27, 2017

My hair finally started falling out. And man, did it fall out. I've been shaving my head with Jon's clippers once a week, so my hair's been short and stubbly, but today in the shower, I noticed all the stubble coming off. As I lathered up, I ran my hand over my skull and those tiny hairs filled my palm. I kept touching my head, and the hairs kept coming off.

OK, time to bust out the Bic razor and channel my inner Dwayne Johnson.

When Jon got home from his gig, I told him we're Bic-ing. And you know what? I wasn't sad. I didn't cry. I didn't mope or have an emotional breakdown. It was fine. He simply shaved my head and at the end, I looked like a hairless cat.

Jon and I took Brian and Anita to the beach. We had a blast. We snapped some adorable group photos along the pier, strolled along the shops, then enjoyed a vegan feast at Gracias Madre. Anita is a doctor, so we chatted about medical stuff, and I loved getting her input on my cancer fiasco. I'm insanely happy that I got to see her and Brian this weekend.

Tuesday, May 30, 2017

I made an appointment to meet my new boob doctor (who happens to be Dr. Li's wife). Her name is Dr. Dang, and I shall refer to her as The Breast Whisperer. The initial consult will probably be a slew of Q&As, but eventually I'll get a mammogram, and I'm sure we'll discuss my double mastectomy. Even though surgery won't happen until later next year, I want all the information now—especially the most important factor: implant size! I'm naturally a 36D, but wouldn't it be fun to get huge watermelon boobs? I want ones that'll hit me in the face when I'm jogging.

I've conducted some research on adopting, and purchasing a kiddo costs a lot of money. Like thirty grand. *Does Bank Of America do Baby Loans?*

And on a frustrating note, I noticed that my short-term memory isn't as sharp as it used to be. I find myself repeating the same story several times without realizing it, until someone gently points out that I'm being redundant, and someone gently points out that I'm being redundant. Haha, just kidding (sort of).

Thursday, June 1, 2017

Today I visited The Dog Cafe, a very cool "halfway house" for rescued dogs that lets you cuddle with puppies while sipping coffee. Heaven. For two hours, I snuggled with a ten-year old blind Chihuahua named Carla. If I were in a better fiscal situation, I would have adopted her on the spot. #bleedingheartproblems

Looking forward to resuming chemo tomorrow. Just wanna get these last few sessions over with so we can proceed with the hysterectomy. It's been two weeks since Chemo Session #5, and my appetite has come back full force. I've been eating a little too much and now I feel fat. All I need is for that hair on my face to grow back, and I can be fat, bald, and hairy. Somehow I've morphed from a cheery thirty-six-year-old woman to a sixty-year-old uncle version of myself.

Friday, June 2, 2017

Yes! Got cleared for chemo after my blood work today, so we knocked out Session #6 and thus completed Cycle #2. My white blood cell count had dipped down to 600 (4,500 to 11,000 is the normal range), but today it was back up to 1600. Whew.

Before treatment, I met with my Rockstar Cancer Ninja Dr. Li and Angelic Nurse Practitioner Corina for a checkup. They're gonna put me on estrogen right after the hysterectomy, which should ease the symptoms caused by menopause (hot flashes, insomnia, anxiety, irritability, moodiness). Dr. Li said lots of women in L.A. take estrogen and refer to it as the "fountain of youth."

Wait, so, I'm losing my ovaries and uterus, but I'll look younger? Sign me up.

Blood clots are a risk with the estrogen pill, and surgery increases the risk of clots, so I'll have to wear an estrogen patch for the first couple of months. That's cool with me, because half the time I forgot to take my birth control pill. I'm actually sort of surprised I never got pregnant.

I've started putting together my Post-Chemo-Vanity-Plan, which includes a tattoo, Botox, Restylane, and spider vein treatment. Dr. Li said everything has to wait until we're finished with chemo. I'm probably putting too much emphasis on my vanity, but it's hard not to when you're bald.

The bills are piling up. Remember those three days I was in the emergency room, when I got my biopsy and met Dr. Li for the first time? That cost $27,000. And one chemo session? That's $10,700, and I'm having eighteen chemo sessions total. And I'm not sure how much the hysterectomy will cost, but I imagine tens of thousands. So in the end, I estimate that ovarian cancer will cost around $400,000. As much as I gripe about insurance, I would literally be dead without it. And because I'm BRCA-positive, insurance will cover the double mastectomy and implants, which should run up another $50-60K. Cancer is expensive. Do you know how much shit I could buy with $400K? By my calculations:

- 16 Toyota Priuses
- 400 rounds of Botox and fillers
- 40 bottles of Pappy Van Winkle's Family Reserve 23-Year-Old Bourbon
- 666 pounds of pule cheese, the most expensive cheese in the world (which comes from Serbian donkeys)
- A billboard on Sunset Blvd for two years featuring my cat
- A teeny condo in Los Angeles with no driveway and cracks in the ceilings

---

Sunday, June 4, 2017

Had a wonderful time catching up with friends this weekend. Saturday I went to lunch with Chrispy, one of my favorite former coworkers from a post-production company. He's a very talented photographer with razor-sharp wit. He used to tease me about the ugly clothes I wore to work, but he was right to do so. I went through a phase where I only wore collared shirts from Express with buckles on the sleeves, and they never quite fit correctly. And don't get me started about what he said when I stupidly wore a sundress with tube socks. Anyway, we met for tacos, and he invited me to his Gay Pride party next weekend. Rainbows, filthy jokes, and the best brunch in the world. Yes, please.

Today I met up with another former coworker, Anne, whom I worked with at a failing tech startup last year. Our cubicles were side-by-side, and we'd take giggle breaks while I ate her homemade kale chips. Anne is smart, down-to-earth, and always rocks a kick-ass hairstyle (today it was a badass blue shag, which looked a lot more natural than the blue pile of yarn resting on my head). We reminisced about the good days, the bad days, and the days where our bosses didn't bother to hide the piles of narcotics in their pockets.

On my way back from lunch, my wig itched, so I took it off and enjoyed the summer breeze on my dome. I parked and hesitated before getting out of the car. What if I ran into a neighbor and they saw my head? I'm so paranoid without a bandana or wig. There's a very short list of people who look good with a bald shiny head (*hi, Vin Diesel*). I hate feeling this way. I scurried through the hallways, clutching my wig, heart beating fast, and exhaled a sigh of relief from the safety of my apartment. I know I need to come to terms with this, so...

I took a selfie of my head, sans wig and sans bandana, and posted it on Facebook and Instagram before I could change my mind. *Crap. Now it's out there for the world to see.* My stomach lurched in fear, and I wanted to take the photo down, but I didn't. And guess what? Nothing bad happened. No one judged me. In fact, dozens of comments immediately poured in, full of kindness and support. Hmmm. I guess that wasn't so bad. And neither was chemo. In fact, nothing has been as scary as I made it out to be in my mind.

Perhaps there's nothing to fear except fear itself?

Monday, June 5, 2017

I had a little nausea this morning, but Zofran took care of that. After the queasiness subsided, a total-body exhaustion knocked me on my ass. Eventually I forced myself to go for a walk under the assumption that some light shopping would awaken my heavy limbs. I bought a cute pair of Converse and a new bed set (which was only

$36, and it'd be stupid to pass on savings like that). Only problem is, I left the store and realized I'd have to lug the huge bags up a hill. For a second I considered calling a Lyft, but catching a ride just three blocks would be too shameful.

I huffed and puffed and shuffled my way back, but had to stop every five feet to adjust the plastic handles digging into my palms. Halfway home, I sought refuge at my favorite coffee shop and plopped down at a patio table, sweaty and depleted. A delicious almond milk latte revived me and gave me the necessary push to drag my ass up the hill.

Knocked out a solid thirty minutes on the elliptical and felt great. I still wanna drop like fifteen more pounds (I think I'm down about twenty to twenty-five since this started). I feel like the people who administer chemo should start advertising weight loss as one of its benefits.

Jon got us tickets to a live taping of a comedy show called *This Is Not Happening*. One of our favorite comics, Bret Ernst, was performing. The show is supposed to air on Comedy Central in 2018, and it was filmed at a Hollywood strip club. As an audience member, I knew there was a chance my face would be on TV, so I applied five layers of makeup and put on my red wig. Once we got to the venue, I caught my reflection and wasn't sure whether I looked like a vivacious comedy-goer or an exotic dancer. The show was absolutely hilarious, but I started to feel sick about halfway through, and realized I left my Zofran at home. Thankfully, the fourteen layers of foundation on my cheeks hid the greenish hue of queasiness.

Tuesday, June 6, 2017

I'm officially back on coffee. I've had a few lattes here and there, but today I got my first iced coffee since the diagnoses. I added a teeny pinch of stevia, although I would have preferred five packs of sugar.

I miss the days of carelessly dumping thirty ounces of artificial carcinogenic sweetener into my caffeine.

I've been struggling with feelings of worthlessness. I'm still waiting for Jill's feedback on my book (Has she not read it? Does she hate it?) and this whole wait-'til-cancer-is-over-to-find-a-job thing is taking a toll on me. I don't feel productive. I need to be contributing. Contributing to my bank account. To my career. To my future.

Although I guess I am contributing to my future by ensuring I'll be around for it, right?

Friday, June 9, 2017

So, Jill doesn't hate my manuscript. She had a few small revisions, but overall she said it's great. Woot woot. I can't believe people like my writing. I guess I know the stories I wrote are mildly entertaining (and terribly embarrassing), but I have a hard time comprehending that anything I create is good. I'm starting to understand why many writers are alcoholics. Poor self-esteem + prose + an endless stream of whiskey = where the magic happens.

Today was Chemo Session #7. Everything went off without a hitch. I wore my curly pink wig (Lacy) and felt fierce. I thought it would be cute to bring a couple of props, so I grabbed a martini glass and cocktail shaker out of my kitchen. Got some great Instagram snaps while I enjoyed a "chemo-tini" (just water in the martini glass, but it looked cool). The nurses giggled when they walked past my bay.

My hemoglobin is getting low, but all my other blood levels are in the "somewhat normal-ish" range. And we got my new tumor marker number...it's down to twenty-two! Great news. Last time we checked it was 150. So the chemo is super effective. Just two more chemo sessions, a quick CT scan, and one final meeting with Rockstar Cancer Ninja Dr. Li before my hysterectomy, which I'm now referring to as "getting spayed."

While Jon and I were in the waiting room, I noticed a weird-looking brochure. The cover said, "Can The Dead Really Live Again?" It totally skeeved me out, and I wondered if Cedars has some sort of Zombie Program going on. Jon said the brochure was a Bible thing, intended to give people comfort, but c'mon, we all know that it's zombie propaganda. I'm gonna be real careful when I go to Cedars now on—after battling cancer, there's *no way* I'm getting taken out by an undead skin muncher.

Sunday, June 10, 2017

Yesterday was filled with friends and laughter. Went for a hike with Elina in the afternoon and realized that my lung capacity could use some improvement. I tried to keep up with our conversation as we skedaddled up the hills, but the lack of oxygen left me gasping and saying "fuck this" a lot.

Later I met Andrea for vegan food at Gracias Madre. I almost cracked and ordered a cocktail while we waited for a table, but I remained vigilant and refrained. A drink would have been so satisfying, but I envisioned the liquor seeping into my tumors and breathing strength into those evil cells. Pass.

Today I went to Kara's. She lives a couple of blocks away, and we recently became homies. For the last several months, I saw her every time I went to Starbucks, and one day I decided to introduce myself. I was drawn to her cheery personality, infectious laugh, and penchant for sparkly makeup. Kara's also got a killer sense of humor, which makes sense because she and her husband TK are comedians. They hosted an afternoon shindig, and I ran into my buddy Mike, whom I hadn't seen in months. We traded cancer quips and griped about politics. I had a couple of pains in my stomach, which could be the chemo working, or just an involuntary reaction to discussing the disaster that makes up our current government.

After seeing so many incredible friends this weekend, I felt totally invigorated. I'm very lucky to have so many quality friendships.

_____

Monday, June 12, 2017

Holy crap, I've literally never been this tired in my life. I got up, fed the cats, and went back to bed. Got up, had some breakfast, then went back to bed. Got up, had a snack, then went back to bed. The cats joined me. All my limbs feel like dead weight. I finally forced myself to get a coffee at four p.m. and drank it in bed. Then went back to sleep.

I hope Jon is OK with getting married in bed.

_____

Wednesday, June 14, 2017

I'm probably not qualified to make this comparison, but pregnancy and chemotherapy seem to have similar side effects. All you want to do is sleep. You get random food cravings. You're moody. You eat an entire jar of pickles like an animal, then pass out for two hours. (I was drunk from all the sodium.) The nausea hasn't been bad, but the exhaustion takes all the wind outta my sails. And the real kicker is the insomnia. Daytime = sleep. Nighttime = tossing and turning and going over every stupid thing that I've ever said in my life. Insomnia and neuroses are a bad mix.

_____

Friday, June 16, 2017

Knocked out Chemo Session #8! I wore a very fun '80s-style getup to add a little flavor. Crazy that I'm almost halfway done. My white blood cells are low again, which means Jon gets to clean the kitty litter box, because my body can't fight off infection. And I can't be around people who cough or sneeze or generally have germs...so basically everyone.

Poor Jon. Today is his birthday, and he sat with me during chemo. What a fun way to ring in your thirty-ninth. Afterwards, we went to Fox & Hounds, a fun pub in Studio City. Our favorite cover band, The Lovelies, was playing, and they're a blast. Some of Jon's buddies were there, and he enjoyed himself (along with Jack Daniels shots and a few Old Fashioneds). I didn't drink and still had a great time.

There's one song that I'm obsessed with ("Don't Look Back In Anger" by Oasis), and I just have to dance whenever The Lovelies play it, so Jon and I busted out our best moves in front of the stage. While we boogied away, he dipped me backward and my wig flew off! Since we were right in front of the stage, everyone saw. Ugh.

For a second, I considered rocking my baldness and dancing without my wig, but paranoia took over and I quickly pulled the pink matted mess back onto my head. It was mildly humiliating, but also super funny, so who cares? I'll probably be one of those seventy-year-old women who gets wasted on Grasshoppers and rips off her hairpiece at family reunions, so this was good practice.

_____

Saturday, June 17, 2017

To continue Jon's birthday festivities, we went to Dan Tana's and had a delectable dinner. I longed for a couple of glasses of champagne but managed to stick to sparkling water. We split a tiramisu for dessert, and I thoroughly enjoyed it, but I probably shouldn't have allowed myself so much sugar. I wore my expensive dark wig, Brigitte. The long brunette sheen made me feel like a pretty pony. But my klutziness kicked in, and I spilled pasta, chicken, and green beans on Brigitte's luscious strands. At least the hair is dark so you couldn't really tell. This is why I can't have nice things.

Tuesday, June 20, 2017

I feel fat. I'm still down about twenty pounds from where I began, but after the tiramisu and onslaught of butter over the weekend, my tummy is poking out more than usual. I can hear it pleading with me. *Get it together, bitch.*

I met The Breast Whisperer, Dr. Dang, and she's just as lovely as her husband. They are truly a brilliant power-couple. We talked about my family history and the BRCA gene mutation. She said today I'd get my first mammogram. In December, I'll have an MRI. Then I can schedule an appointment with a reconstructive plastic surgeon to discuss my mastectomy (which will happen in 2018). It's tempting to think about getting huge knockers, but I should probably stick to my current size to avoid back problems.

The mammogram was easy, albeit uncomfortable. You're standing up on your tippy toes, then they smoosh your breast tissue all flat and tell you to hold your breath while they take the x-ray. My poor gals. They did not like being flattened into busty little pancakes. Thankfully, everything looked normal, and there's no cancer in my bosom.

Wednesday, June 21, 2017

I tried Reiki for the first time. My brother Rob swears by it and I was curious to see what it entailed. He thought it might help my mindset, and at this point I'm open to anything. From what I understand, Reiki is an ancient healing technique where the practitioner channels "life force energy" to another person through their hands. #shrug

I found a gal online who seemed cool, and right away I dug her energy and pricing (she only charges $50 per session, while the others I found charged $75 or more). And I loved her potty mouth—she dropped more F-bombs in an hour than I normally do in a whole day. Our session consisted of me lying on a massage-like table while she chanted and occasionally placed her hands on my body. At one point, I almost fell asleep. But mostly I was stuck in my head.

Am I breathing too loud? My checking account is pathetic. Why can't I shut off my stupid brain?

It's like my psyche is stuck on spin cycle, with a pile of worry and anxiety tumbling around, but the mental laundry is never finished. Rob says if I meditate consistently, I'll get a better handle on this. I've been trying to meditate before bed every night, but some nights I don't get around to it. It's kind of like kale—you know it's good for you, but sometimes you can't bother.

Friday, June 23, 2017

Chemo Session #9 like a boss! White blood cells were still low, but high enough that we could do treatment today. I wore my blue wig and for some reason brought a pineapple. I'm not sure why. I think maybe because pineapples are such a happy fruit—they're tasty, attractive, and bring people joy. My nurse snickered.

I'm thrilled to be done with the first half of chemo treatments. They've gone by quickly, and I hope I'll sail through the next half just as smoothly. Apparently the new treatment will be rougher in terms of nausea and exhaustion. We'll be swapping the Carboplatin for another drug called Cisplatin, and it'll be administered directly into my tummy, which sends a concentrated dose directly to the cancer cells. Eek!

I'm psyching myself up for surgery, which is only a week and a half away. Not too nervous, but still very apprehensive about waking up under anesthesia. Dad says there's no way that will happen, and I'm ridiculous to think about it, but it totally happens. I've seen the horror stories on one of those *Some-Scary-Shit-Happened-To-*

Me-And-It-Will-Happen-To-You-Too TV shows. One lady woke up during her operation but couldn't move or speak because of the anesthesia, but she could feel them cutting into her body, and now she can't sleep and suffers from PTSD.

Next week should be exciting—CT scan on Wednesday, then Dr. Li on Friday to review the results and discuss what type of surgery we'll proceed with. There's an easy way (laparoscopically, which means they make a few tiny incisions and remove the organs) and a more invasive way (through my abdomen, with a huge vertical incision and much longer recovery time). Obviously hoping for the easy way, but we shall see—it depends on the CT scan and how small the tumors are. If I don't lose at least two pounds from removing my ovaries and uterus, I'm gonna be pissed. What's the point of surgery if it's not making me skinnier?

Sunday, June 25, 2017

Last night Jon and I went to The Comedy Store. The lineup was spectacular, and it felt great to laugh. We saw Richi (our boxing coach) for the first time in months (he's a General Manager there), and I allowed myself two cocktails. And they tasted outstanding. I'm harboring a little guilt because I know sugar is my arch nemesis right now, but I figured, hey, I just powered through nine chemo sessions, and I deserve a little indulgence (I mean, Dr. Li *did* say I could still live my life and have treats in moderation). I just hope the tumors aren't sitting in my belly being like, "HELL YEAH! SUGAR! LET'S METASTASIZE, MOTHERFUCKERS!"

Had lunch with Ty, a coworker from when I waited tables circa 2013. Ty's got a solid sense of humor (he often made obscene gestures from behind the bar, when customers couldn't see him) and... he's also bald! This was the first time I'd seen him since I started chemo, and even though he's a fellow member of The Baldie Club,

I didn't have the confidence to rock my hairless dome in public. We went to a Mexican joint, and cocktails were included with the price of brunch, but I passed and just drank water…and salsa. Yes, you can drink salsa.

Jill said my book is "pitch-ready" and she's gonna start reaching out to major publishing houses. I'm *so* hoping to score a book deal but trying to keep my expectations in check. Being able to call myself an "author" on something besides my blog would be a true Bucket List checkmark. And it'd shine such a happy light onto an otherwise dark and cancer-y period in my life.

Kim Tronic—author, cancer survivor, and literary floozy.

———————

Tuesday, June 27, 2017

My eyebrows have been hanging on for dear life, but I think it's time to give in and pluck off the last few stragglers. Up until now, I've been protective of every little strand up there, but it's finally at the point where no hair will look better than a couple of sad dawdlers. Grabbed my tweezers and off they went. Now I *really* look like a cancer patient, and it's not cute.

I don't know why, but tonight I said a prayer before bed. I'm not a particularly religious person (my dad is Jewish and my mom is Protestant), and prayer always felt weird to me. I never went to church, so I felt like a fraud if I tried to converse with God. Like, *Hey God, I can't be bothered to worship you once a week before getting drunk at Sunday brunch, but can you do me a super huge favor? Cool, thanks God, good lookin' out, Bro.* Plus, when I hear people spew intolerance toward homosexuals, transgenders, or abortion, they tend to lean on the Bible and its rhetoric, so religion in the "traditional" sense hasn't appealed to me. My religion is more along the lines of, *Be a good person. Be kind. Be empathetic. Accept others. Don't be an asshole. Wash your hands. And for fuck's sake, leave the toilet seat down.* But for some reason, tonight I felt the urge to say wassup to God. We had a short conversation (it was very one-sided), and it felt weird and uncomfortable, like when you have a giant wedgie in public, and you can't pick it.

Wednesday, June 28, 2017

CT scan today. Had to drink a horribly disgusting mocha-flavored paste. It was warm, milky, and murky. I literally gagged six times. It tasted like a latte that had been left out in the sun for a couple of days, then got blended with cyanide and mayonnaise. The scan itself was quick. As I moved back and forth through the huge machine, I had to wonder what my tumors look like. Are they teeny brown lumps? Puffy white algae?

I totally spaced on planning my Farewell Uterus party. But that's OK because Friday I'm going out with Ashley and friends, and we'll give my organs a nice send off. Jon ordered a sheet cake with "See Ya Later, Ovulator!" spelled out in frosting. How thoughtful is that?

Reconnected with a few of my coworkers from my last job (the startup that kicked me to the curb). Jake got a great new job at another startup, and I'm happy for him. He's such a smarty-pants, and he'll kick some major ass at the new venture. I had lunch with Jamie, the adorable intern. She just got back from an incredible vacation where she visited Croatia and Budapest. Super jealous! She showed me pics of her drinking cocktails, riding bikes, and swimming in dazzling clear oceans. She's moving up north to San Francisco next week, so I'm glad we got to hang before she takes off. I got an email from Amy, one of the heads of the company (she's still there) and we made plans to grab coffee. I'm grateful to be in touch with these wonderful homies despite the scattered roads we're all on.

Friday, June 30, 2017

Met with Rockstar Cancer Ninja Dr. Li to review the CT scan and discuss next week's surgery. He's encouraged by how much my tumors have shrunk, but the tumors on my spleen ruined its blood supply so we need to remove it. To access the area, we have to go with the invasive procedure. I'll stay in the hospital for a few days, and recovery should take about four weeks. While my belly is open, Dr. Li will put in a passport (to administer the chemo treatments going forward) as well as two catheters (to directly infuse pain medication). Ugh. I'm anticipating a lot of discomfort in my future.

Also, since I won't have a spleen, I'll need to get certain vaccines for the rest of my life. Apparently one is for pneumonia, one is for some weird strain of the flu, and one is for meningitis. Not a huge deal, but a little irritating. Next week I can stop taking the birth control pill, and I'll start estrogen the day of surgery. I'll have a patch on, but eventually I can switch to a daily estrogen pill. Curious to see how much that will help with the side effects from menopause. If I grow a mustache, I'm gonna be so mad. (Although, I already had a beard, so surely a mustache wouldn't be much worse. I might even look smart and distinguished.)

Dr. Li said I'll definitely be in remission after surgery and remaining chemo treatments. It's great to hear that from the Jedi Cancer Master himself. I'm trying to focus on that, and not let my fear of waking up under anesthesia take over my psyche.

To celebrate, Jon and I had dinner with Ashley and friends at Hamburger Mary's. Seriously, if you ever need a self-esteem boost, go here. The handsome, sassy servers dish up endless compliments (and insults, if you can handle it), and you always leave smiling. Our server gave me a huge sparkling water with mint and limes to make me feel like part of the drinking crowd. And he put two giant fiery sparkler candles on my "See Ya Later, Ovulator!" cake. I felt loved and supported. And super fat after I had four pieces of cake.

Monday, July 3, 2017

OK, now I'm getting nervous for surgery. Logically, I know it will go smoothly and I'm in the best possible hands. But I'm scared of the pain and the aftermath. Mom and Dad will fly out this Sunday because they don't want me being alone next week while Jon's at work. I'm happy I'll get to see them, but I feel bad they'll just be sitting at my apartment while I'm crabby and living in a medication-induced haze. I would rather have them out here when I'm healthier and able to walk around the city. However, I understand that something could go wrong during recovery, and it would behoove me to have people around for the first couple of weeks.

Jon took me out for a super bomb BBQ dinner. I treated it like my last meal before I get spayed. Technically tomorrow night is the last meal, but tomorrow I wanna eat light because I don't want any tummy discomfort (aka have an involuntary toot) during the procedure. How embarrassing would that be? I mean, OK, I won't actually *know* if I pass gas under anesthesia. But everyone else will know. And Dr. Li is strikingly handsome, so I can't be coma-tooting in his holy presence.

Or, what if they're in the middle of operating near my nether region, and a toot slips out, and all those fart particles (farticles?) contaminate the air and they have to shut down the ER because of my flatulence? *Do other people worry about this?*

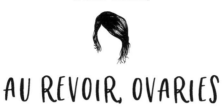

PART THREE

AU REVOIR, OVARIES

Tuesday, July 4, 2017

Holy crap, I can't believe surgery is tomorrow. I spent today the best way I knew how: shopping and cleaning. Got three new colorful wigs: green (affectionately named Medusa), hot pink (Polly), and rainbow (Rainbow Brite). Then went into a gorgeous boutique and fell in love with their quirky merchandise. The tops had ruffles, the pants had mesh cutouts, and the dresses were slinky and funky. One little black number with white polka dots and a huge embroidered rose fit me like a glove. I bought it 'cuz sometimes a bitch gotta treat herself.

After my shopping spree, Jon and I got manicures and pedicures. I wanna look as pretty as possible while I'm drooling on myself at the hospital. I frittered away the evening with laundry, a quick workout, and tidying the apartment. I probably packed too much for my jaunt at Cedars. Mostly I'll be in a gown, but what if they let me change, and I want options? Better to over pack than under pack. Plus, Cedars has been known to treat celebrities (well, to deliver their babies anyways), and what if there's paparazzi wandering the halls? I'd hate to be in a wrinkly hospital gown for my tabloid debut.

Wednesday, July 5, 2017

Barely slept last night. The anxiety was killing me. I've never had major surgery like this, and I kept tossing and turning as my mind explored every worst case scenario: too much anesthesia, not enough anesthesia, brain damage, and of course…death.

I woke up at the crack of dawn, hopped into the shower, and Jon drove us to Cedars. We checked in with reception and waited to get called for sign-in and paperwork. A nervous energy filled the room, and I met eyes with a couple of other patients. I think we all felt that same jittery anticipation.

They brought me into a frigid room where you undress, wipe down your entire body with sterile cloths, put on a gown, and cover your head with a sterile cap. I huddled on my bed, cold, vulnerable, and scared. A very nice nurse came by and asked a bunch of questions, and I signed a few forms. Then my anesthesiologist introduced himself and assured me I wouldn't wake up on the table. He said to stop watching so much TV (*fine, Dad, you're right this one time*) and started my IV. The drug kicked in immediately, and I felt drowsy and suddenly didn't have a care in the world. I got to see Jon for a quick second, and apparently he snapped a few selfies of us, which I don't remember. They wheeled me into the operating room and I recall making a few jokes, then everything went black.

Holy. Fucking. Shit.

I woke up to a brutal stabbing sensation across my entire midsection. The pain was absolutely excruciating, but I was too weak to cry, so I whimpered. Someone wheeled my bed up to the eighth floor and put me in a room where I'd reside for the next few days. As they lifted me onto my new bed, the pain multiplied and it took my breath away. The rest of the day was a haze, and my throat was killing me (presumably from the intubation). And for some reason, I wasn't allowed to drink water, so I couldn't speak (which must have been a nice change for Jon). I had to whisper when I needed anything.

I was heavily sedated, but the pain snuck through and burned my insides. As bedtime approached, the nurse put "leg squeezers" on me, which are a modern day torture device. They inflate with air, then deflate, then inflate again, then deflate again. It may sound nice, but imagine trying to sleep while someone systematically grabs your legs four times a minute. The squeezers prevent blood clots, but I could only sleep in twenty-minute increments. It was not a pleasant evening.

Thursday, July 6, 2017

Thank God I could drink water today. The inside of my mouth was like sawdust. All morning I greedily gulped down water like a dehydrated desert nomad.

They took my catheter out, so now I have to shuffle to the bathroom for potty breaks. It's only a three-foot journey, but it feels like fifty. When I'm lying down and pull myself into a sitting position, searing pain shoots across my belly and I collapse. Then I have to pause, recuperate, and muster the strength to pull myself into a standing position. I never knew that simply using the potty could be such a monstrous hassle.

Rockstar Cancer Ninja Dr. Li said surgery went well and my stomach looks great. I can't bring myself to look at my belly, but apparently the scar is covered by a bandage. There's also a new passport inside my lower right tummy and an estrogen patch stuck to my skin. Total chaos down there. I want no part of it. I'll just pretend my lower body doesn't exist.

Jon spent the day by my side, and we watched Netflix. I received some beautiful flowers, one bouquet from Mom and Dad, one from my sweet in-laws. Everyone on social media has been really supportive, and I love reading the comments and messages. Mom and Dad are coming to visit on Sunday.

As much as I love Cedars, I wanna get out of here. I never thought I would spend this much time in a hospital.

Friday, July 7, 2017

I officially hate the bathroom. It's just too painful getting in and out of bed for potty breaks, so now I hang out in a chair by my window, which has a gorgeous view of Los Angeles.

Cedars lost power around two in the afternoon. Jon and I were walking in the hallway, and we suddenly got plunged into total darkness. Turns out the whole block lost power, and it didn't come back on until four a.m. Which means no TV and no air conditioning for fourteen hours. Cedars does have a back-up generator, but that only keeps power for emergency services, like operating room equipment. I felt terrible for the hospital staff, who had to bear the brunt of complaining patients. Thankfully my room stayed relatively cool—until I tried to sleep.

After Jon went home, it was quiet. Too quiet. Since there was no AC blowing through the vents and no TV playing in anyone's room, a heavy silence filled the hallways. It was creepy. Hospitals are a prime location for horror movies, and I have a very active imagination.

Jon left me his iPad, so I watched a few comedy specials on Netflix to keep my mind in a positive place. I nodded off for a couple of hours in bed, then a nurse woke me up for vitals. I was covered in sweat. After she departed, I tried to sleep on the couch, because the cushions were made of vinyl and felt much cooler than my clammy sheets. I dozed for a few more hours and was awakened again for vitals. By this time, the power had come back on and I could hear the happy whoosh of the AC. Finally! When I got up from the couch, my stomach was stuck to the cushions, and I had to peel my tummy off the vinyl very carefully without ripping my bandages.

Saturday, July 8, 2017

SO HAPPY TO BE HOME.

It took a while to get my medications and discharge instructions, so we didn't check out until mid-afternoon.

I have Norco and Ibuprofen for pain. I'll have to give myself an injection of blood thinner each day for the next couple of weeks to prevent blood clots. The nurse showed me how to pinch my tummy fat (plenty to choose from) then plunge the medicine right into my skin. It hurts. A huge bruise developed there later in the day. I also took home a few estrogen patches, which I adhere to my lower abdomen and switch out once a week. Hopefully this will prevent hot flashes and insomnia. Can't believe I'm officially a member of the Menopause Club.

Does this mean I qualify for the AARP and discounted movie tickets?

I'm still super swollen and gross. Oh, did I mention that I'm wearing a medical girdle? Sexy. I accidentally caught a glimpse of my surgery scar, and it's heinous and long and angry and purple. It starts right under my breasts and snakes all the way down to my crotch, surrounded by a gigantic dark bruise. Purple is my favorite color, but seeing so many hues spattered across my belly makes me rethink its beauty.

Sunday, July 9, 2017

Mom and Dad arrive today! They get in around eight p.m., so I won't see them until tomorrow. I'm trying to clean my apartment, which is unnecessary because I know they won't judge me, but they never stop being your parents, and I want them to be proud of my tidiness.

I slept on the couch last night because my bed is raised off the ground, and there's no way I can pull myself in and out. I was really cold as I fell asleep, but I woke up covered in sweat at four a.m. I had to prop myself up to peel off my sweatshirt, but the pain made it nearly impossible. I eventually knocked back out after struggling to find a comfortable position.

I walked on the treadmill for fifteen minutes and did some light leg stretches. It looks like the swelling is going down a bit, but everything is still kinda huge. I wish the bloating would subside. After all, what's the point of removing your organs if you don't feel skinny afterwards?

Monday, July 10, 2017

Had a great day with my parents. They came to my place and we watched some delicious reruns. I was pleased to discover that Dad enjoys *Botched*, one of my favorite shows. And Mom likes *Catfish* ("That Nev is just so cute!"), so my folks have great taste in reality TV (though Mom will vehemently deny she watches it).

They carted me around for errands, and I feel bad that they're basically my executive assistants. I know this is what they came out for, but I feel guilty. *Can I put them on payroll?*

Dad keeps saying I'm recovering much faster than he anticipated—he thought I'd still be bedridden and suffering. I did, too. Mom and I walked on the treadmill for a bit, and I'm thrilled to exercise. But then I tried to be a hero and vacuum my apartment—big mistake. I got lightheaded and dizzy and almost vomited. It's also kind of hard to get in a full satisfying deep breath. But hey, breathing is overrated, right?

Thursday, July 13, 2017

Tonight we ventured out to one of my all-time favorite restaurants, Musso & Frank's. Dad totally got a kick out of the classic décor and "old Hollywood" charisma. The sassy handsome bartender was chock full of Brooklyn attitude, and kept calling my mom "Bella." We got to sit in Frank Sinatra's booth.

I wore the sexy Brigitte wig so Dad could see his million dollars were well spent. He kept raving about how good it looked, and I think he realized you can't put a price on self-esteem. Speaking of which, when will my hair grow back? I haven't had chemo in almost a month, and my head is still bald and stubbly. *Wait, what if my hair never grows back and I'm bald forever?* On social media, I pretend I'm embracing my baldness and use hashtags like #baldielocks and #baldisthenewblack, but really I'm fucking miserable without hair.

Saturday, July 15, 2017

Yesterday I took Mom and Dad to the wax museum. It's only a few blocks from my apartment, but it's also such a touristy thing to do that I'd probably never go there left to my own devices. It was a hoot! The wax figures were so realistic that a few times I wondered if a real celebrity was posing as their own statue. Dad took pictures with Jack Nicholson and Moses. I posed with ET and Marilyn Monroe. We grabbed lunch at Hard Rock Cafe afterwards and laughed at our ridiculous photos.

Today we went to Ripley's Believe It Or Not museum, which is also a short walk from my apartment. It did not go as well as the wax museum. Once we got downstairs to peruse the oddities in the basement, the air felt thick and wet. I snuck a glance at the thermostat— eighty-three degrees. I suddenly felt queasy and had to sit down immediately. Luckily there was a small room with a few benches, and I gratefully plopped down. Mom and Dad freaked out and insisted we leave, so we zipped out of there and went to lunch. We trudged to Hard Rock Cafe, and the air conditioning brought instant relief. Even though I feel decent most of the time, my body is still recovering, and I should probably slow down and respect the journey.

Tuesday, July 18, 2017

Had my follow up with Rockstar Cancer Ninja Dr. Li this morning. He said my scar is healing perfectly, and we can resume chemo a week from Friday, on July 28th. He said the head rushes and dizziness I'm experiencing are due to anemia. Huh. I can start incorporating small bouts of jogging into my walks and begin lifting weights in a couple of weeks. They gave me three vaccinations since my spleen is gone. And Dr. Li prescribed a smaller estrogen patch. The one I'm wearing now is huge. Jon calls it my granny patch.

The last couple of days I've been struggling with some emotional quirkiness, or as I like to call it, when my mind gets "itchy." It happens when I have too much time on my hands, when I have too much time to think, and I begin to hate everything. I hate my apartment. It feels messy and claustrophobic. I hate my body. It's pale and veiny and I feel old and ugly. I feel like I have no purpose. Dr. Li helps people all day, every day, then goes home to his loving wife and children, and what do I do? Sit around all day and accomplish nothing. It's like life is passing me by, and I'm not living it to the fullest. I know this shit is only temporary, but my cabin fever is beginning to chip away at every shred of happiness in my body. I'm essentially a human slug, capable of nothing but eating and sleeping and complaining and crying.

Sunday, July 23, 2017

Oh God. This week has been an emotional disaster. Everything made me cry. TV commercials. Billboards. My own reflection. A couple of times I felt so sad, so downtrodden and depressed that I could barely force myself to leave the apartment. Dark thoughts kept swirling around my head. *Will I ever get a job again? Should*

I consider an entirely new career path? Will I ever own a house? Get married? What can I do to help save the planet? Will I ever feel totally happy and fulfilled?

After a few days of constant crying, I wondered where this emotional explosion came from. *Had I unknowingly shoved my negative thoughts and feelings down into a pit, and now they were floating to the surface? In my quest to remain happy and positive, had I draped myself under a smiling giggly facade that was now falling away?*

A proverbial light bulb suddenly switched on. Duh. *Welcome to menopause, motherfucker.* I can't believe this didn't occur to me earlier. A bunch of organs have been removed, and I'm wearing an estrogen patch. My hormones have no idea what's going on, so I'm a hyper-sensitive little wreck.

Monday, July 24, 2017

Feeling way more positive. Saw Kara (my comedian neighbor) yesterday and mingled with lots of cool people at her house. I also ate lots of cheese; pepper jack, goat, cheddar, colby...you name it. It was dairy heaven. Even if I get constipated for a week, it was worth it. *Is cheese the missing link to my happiness?*

I'm psyched to resume chemo this Friday—the sooner I start, the sooner I finish. Friday will be Taxol in my arm, Saturday will be Cisplatin in my tummy, and the next couple of days I'll go back in for IV fluid hydration. The hydration seems silly to me—can't I just promise to drink eight gallons of water to flush my kidneys?

Over the weekend, Jon and I visited Hollywood Costume shop to get fun props for chemo, so I hope my nurses are prepared for Luau Day (hello, coconut bra), for Mardi Gras Day (beads, anyone?) and for Gangster Day (yes, I bought a gold grill for my teeth).

Tuesday, July 25, 2017

I thought I was going to die today.

Last time I went to the pot store to stock up on cannabis oils, they only had the "activated" formula. Normally I buy the non-psycho-active oils, which means there's no high, but this time I just grabbed what they had and figured I wouldn't have any issues.

I was wrong.

I was in the middle of cutting up vegetables when I started to feel weird. A major haze was setting in and I felt cloudy. OMG. No. I was not prepared for this. My heart started racing, and I panicked.

Fuck. My heart is on the verge of exploding.

Oh, wait. I remembered that I'd unintentionally had like four servings of double-strength espresso earlier, thinking it was normal coffee, so that accounts for the rapid pulse. OK, cool. And this hor-rible stoned feeling is because of the stupid activated cannabis oil. *Whew. Maybe I won't die today. But my poor body has already endured so much, will I be able to survive this stress on my heart? Maybe I should meditate. But after I call 911?*

Meditating totally helped. Within ten minutes, my pulse returned to normal. I will never take that activated cannabis oil again...or drink that much espresso in a sitting. I was honestly two minutes away from calling an ambulance. How embarrassing would that have been?

"Uh hi, I think I'm dying. I took some weed oil and drank too much coffee. Can you please make sure my heart doesn't fail? Better bring the paddles and a stretcher, just in case. And some Cheetos."

Friday, July 28, 2017

Chemo Session #10! First day back after surgery and only eight more treatments after today. Finally feels like we're inching toward the end. It was only Taxol in my arm IV, so I knew the drill. Taxol days tend to be four to five hours (depending on how quickly the lab can process my blood work before we begin). Double-Dipper days (Taxol plus Cisplatin) can take up to eight hours. I really need to send a fruit basket to the dude who invented Netflix—chemo would be unbearable without my incessant binge-watching.

I wore my Hawaiian-themed costume and was pretty proud. I sported a flower lei necklace, coconut bra, and green wig (Medusa). Treatment went smoothly, but I'm nervous for tomorrow. It'll be my first time getting Cisplatin and my first time utilizing the stomach port. I know in theory everything should be fine, but I'm uneasy about the idea of an IV pumping drugs into my precious belly. My tummy's already been through a lot—it shouldn't have to be pillaged by an onslaught of chemo poison.

My nurse today warned me that Cisplatin's side effects will be difficult to handle—apparently Cisplatin is known as Carboplatin's evil stepsister—but since I'm young and strong I should be able to handle it. However, I studied the look in her eye, and it seemed to say, "Girl, brace yourself."

Saturday, July 29, 2017

Chemo Session #11. Had one of my favorite nurses today, Cindy Kim. I took it as a good sign that her last name matches my first. She assured me she's an expert at doing the tummy IV (which is called Intraperitoneal chemotherapy). It wasn't that painful getting the needle inserted, but once the needle was in, I wasn't allowed to get out of bed until treatment was done.

I was like, *Uhhh what if I have to pee?*

They're like, *Use a bedpan.*

Ew.

I made sure to use the restroom right before she inserted the needle. I've made it thirty-six years without using a bedpan, and I'll be damned if I'm going to start now. I wore my pink wig (Polly) and donned a princess costume, complete with sparkly tiara and scepter. Princess Tronic rockin' out chemo.

Treatment took forever. First we waited to get my blood results. Then Cindy administered the pre-meds, then fluids (which were double the normal amount), then chemo, then another bag of fluids, then I had to lie on my side (to let the drugs seep throughout my belly), then flip to the other side, then lie on both sides again.

Longest. Day. Ever.

Cindy said I'm gonna feel like crap this week. Thank goodness I refilled my Zofran prescription to ward off the nausea. And I have to come back here for IV fluids tomorrow and the next day. Gah. I love Cedars and all, but being at the hospital four days in a row sounds like a special kind of agony.

Sunday, July 30, 2017

SOS. Send help.

This is by far the worst nausea of my life. It's a good thing I can't get pregnant, because I'll never be able to endure this level of sickness again.

I seriously considered calling Cedars and telling them I couldn't make it for fluids today. The thought of getting into the car, driving over, shuffling to the chemo ward, and sitting with an IV in my arm for three hours seemed impossible. But I had to go. I let Jon drag my corpse out of bed and I sobbed in the car. *Sobbed.* Like a child. My emotions got the best of me and I cried and cried and cried. This was just too hard. My mental grit could only carry me so far, and I wanted to give up.

Poor Jon. Whenever I cry, he cries. I wish our emotional breakdowns could be mutually exclusive, but it seems my meltdowns are contagious.

Once the fluids started flowing, the nausea slowly subsided and I regained control. God. *I just resumed treatment, and I'm this messed up?* This doesn't bode well for the next couple of months. Oh, and I fucking hate food. I can't even look at those disgusting turkey sandwiches that I loved so dearly once upon a yester-month. At least I still have Netflix. Reading and daytime TV aren't distracting enough when I'm at the hospital. I need high quality entertainment. Scoured Craigslist forums looking for a jester.

Monday, July 31, 2017

Today was just as brutal as yesterday. No, actually, it was worse. I took a Zofran the second I woke up, and Jon left to get coffee. That horrible "I'm about to puke" feeling crawled up my throat and I dry heaved a few times, then barfed. I threw up the medication I'd just taken along with the accompanying orange Vitamin Water. At least the toilet bowl turned a nice shade of tangerine. When Jon came back I was splayed across the bath mat like a limp rag.

Cried again on my way to Cedars. It's amusing that crying is my natural reaction to feeling this shitty. Like, everyone keeps saying how strong and inspirational I am, but I'm sobbing hysterically in a rainbow wig. By the time I sat down for fluids, my eyes were puffy and red, and I lied and told my nurse it was allergies. I just couldn't admit that I'm a big baby.

Wednesday, August 2, 2017

I. Despise. Food. Jon made a grilled cheese sandwich for dinner yesterday, and I had to tie a bandana around my face so I couldn't smell it. There's a long list of foods that seem poisonous to me now, and that includes butter, garlic, coffee, chocolate, and everything that's not fruit. Watermelon is my only ally.

I'm noticing some hideous side effects that make me feel like a grotesque troll. Blue veins are popping up everywhere on my legs.

Not little spider veins (which can easily be removed, which I'm planning to do once chemo is done). No, these are active, healthy blue veins that are branching across my precious pale skin, and make me feel like an old lady. I'm ugly. There's nothing that can be done except get a tan.

Also, I started to see these tiny black dots across my entire stomach...which are hair follicles. For some reason, the chemo is empowering these gross follicles to stand up and scream for attention. So my whole tummy is dotted with little black specks. And now I feel like a monster.

Fuck you, Cisplatin. And fuck you, cancer.

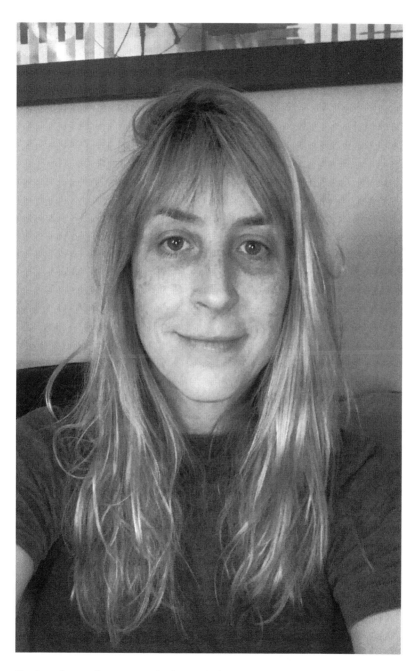

The day after my diagnosis, not looking or feeling my best.

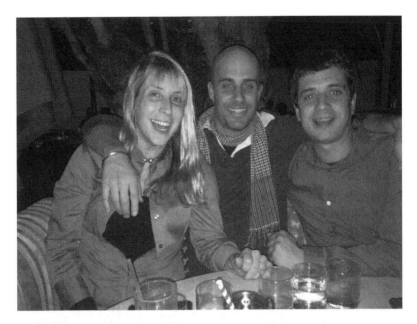

My brothers and I trying to pretend we weren't scared shitless.

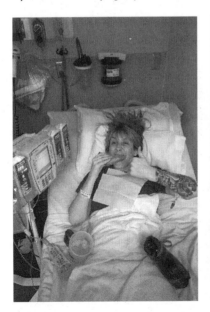

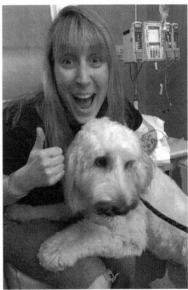

(From left) First and second chemo treatment. Still psyched for free turkey sandwiches.
(Opposite page) Jon and I freshly shorn. And very uncomfortable.

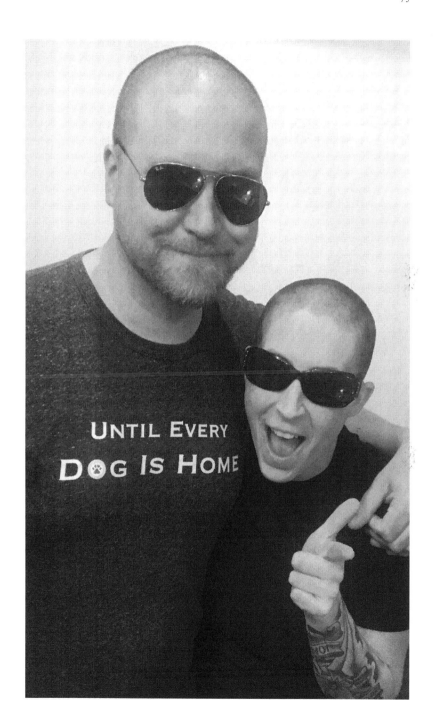

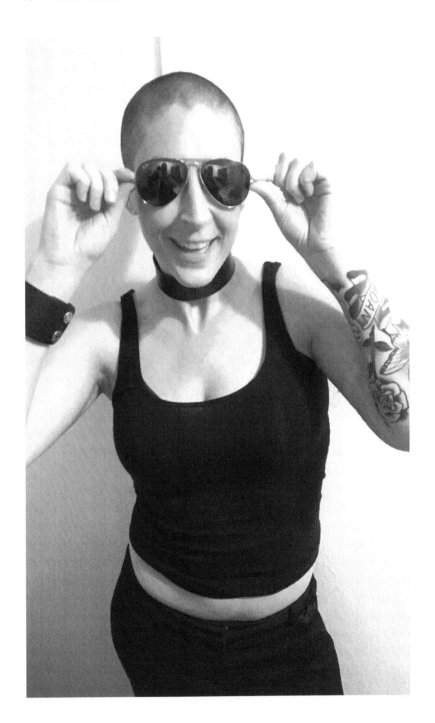

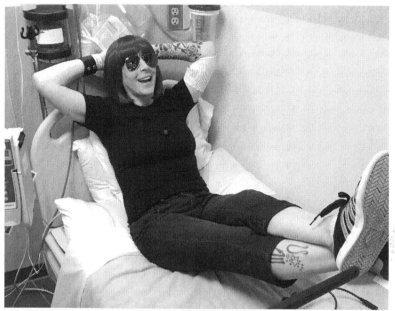

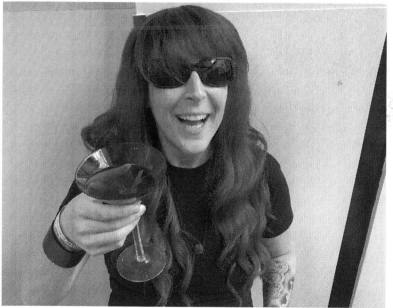

(This page from top) Kickin' back at treatment (chemo #6). Chemo-tini anyone? (chemo #7). (Opposite page) Cancer patient ... or star from *The Matrix?*

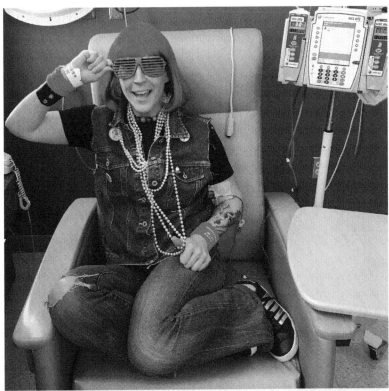

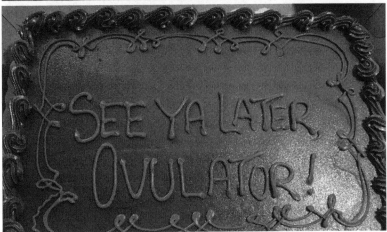

(From top) Pearls and wigs—Grandma would be so proud (chemo #8). Chocolate cake solves all problems. (Opposite page) Having a great hair day.

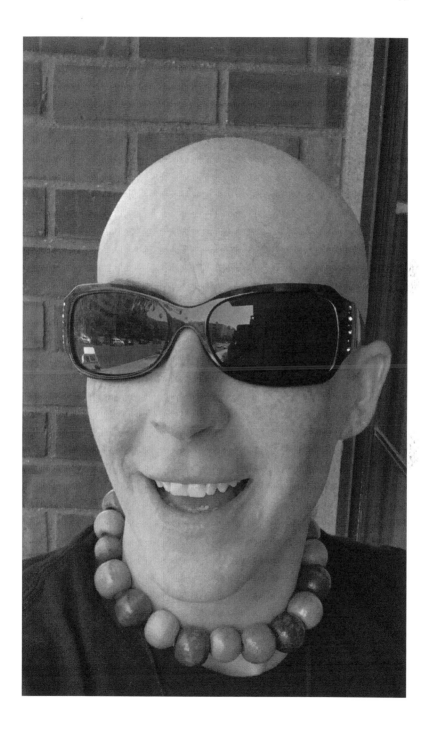

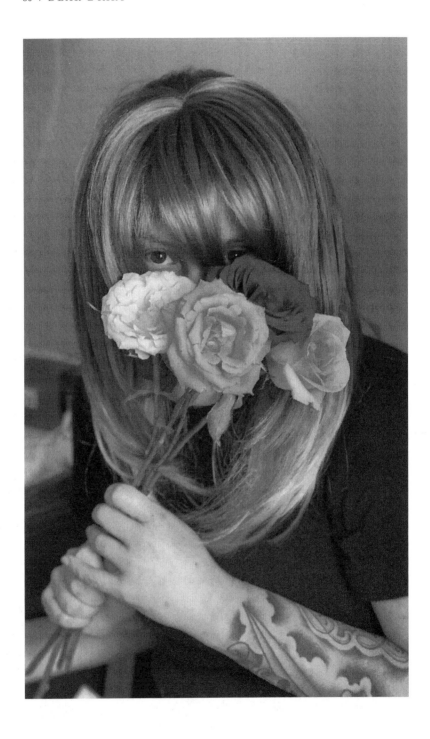

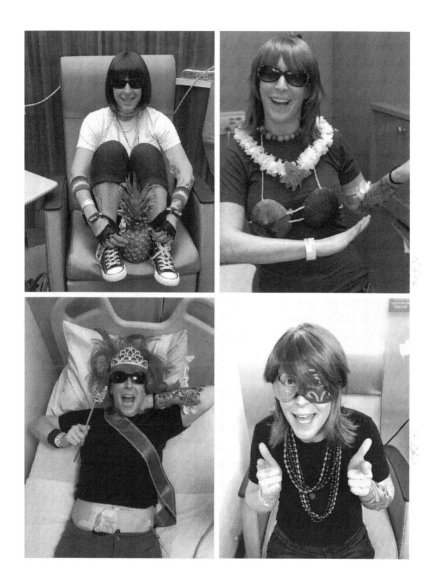

(This page clockwise from top) Chemo costume mashup: Pineapple Day (chemo #9), Luau Day (chemo #10), Princess Day (chemo #11), Mardi Gras Day (chemo #12). (Opposite page) Post-hysterectomy when everything came up roses.

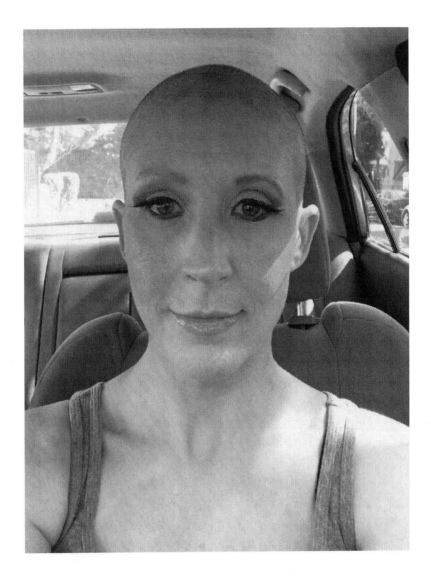

(This page) Does this makeup make me look bald?
(Opposite page) At Kara's anniversary party, thrilled to be in public.

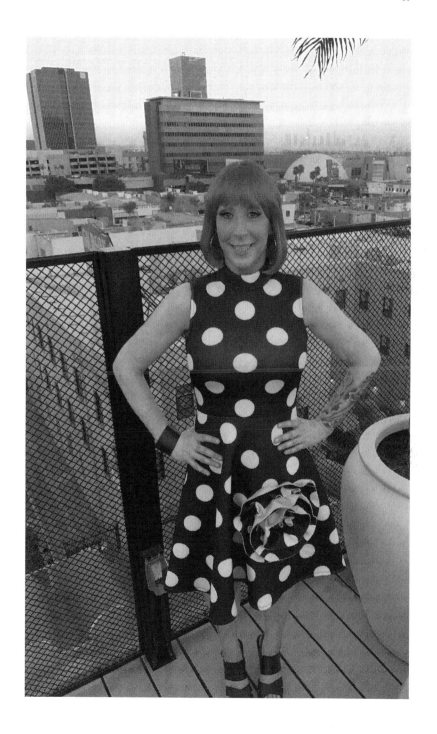

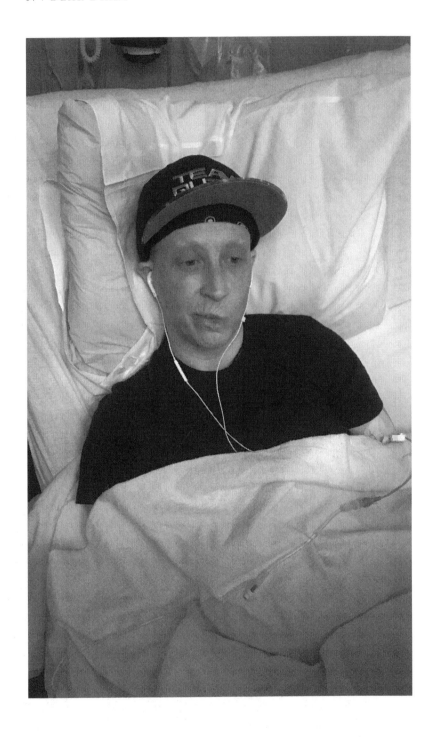

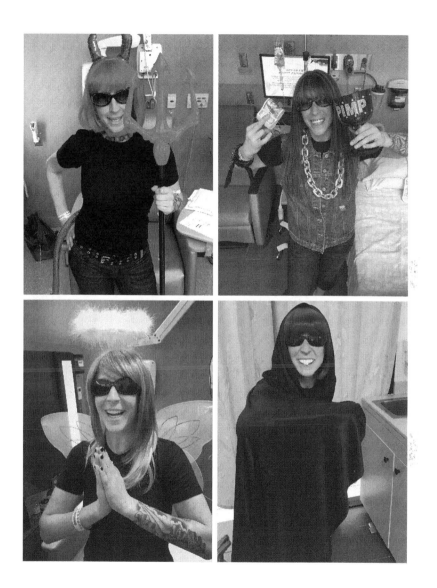

(Clockwise from top left) Chemo costume mashup: Devil Day (chemo #13), Pimp Day (chemo #14), Angel Day (chemo #16), Bucktooth Vampire Day (chemo #17). (Opposite page) Queasy at fluid hydration and less than excited about life.

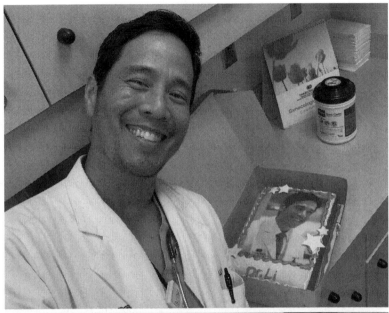

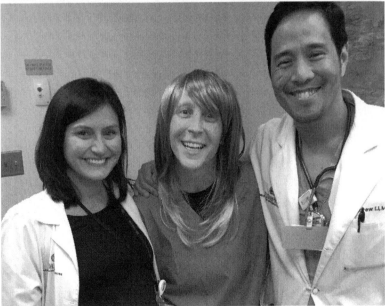

My final chemo treatment with Rockstar Cancer Ninja Dr. Li and
Angelic Nurse Practitioner Corina. (Opposite page) Zen vibes in Sedona.

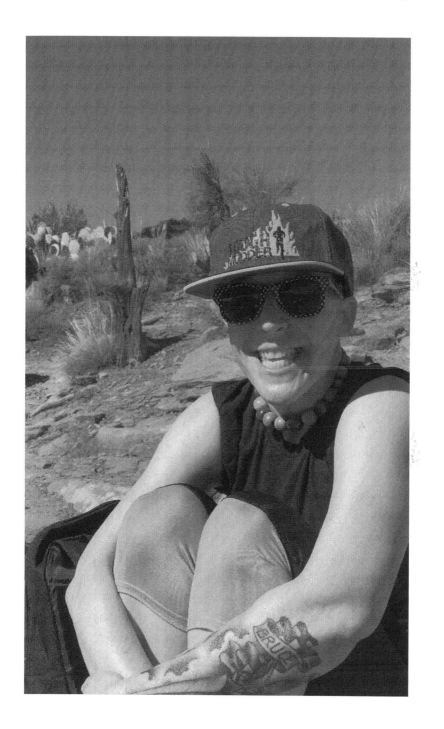

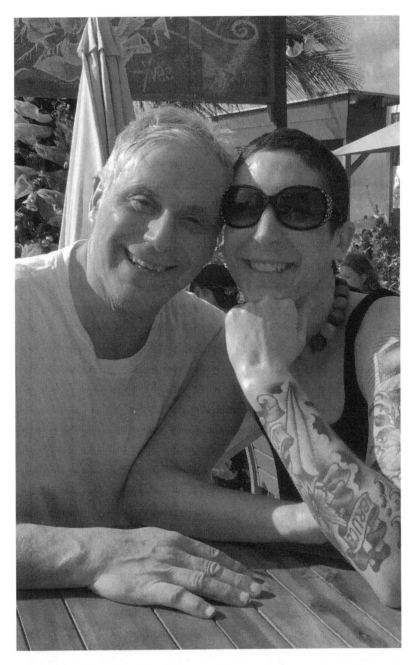

Victory holiday vacation with Dad after a rough year.

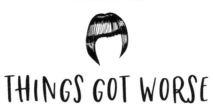

PART FOUR

THINGS GOT WORSE

Thursday, August 3, 2017

Went to see Mahankirn (my energy healer) for a Sat Nam Rasayan appointment. I was so queasy this morning I debated canceling, but figured I should power through and get some much-needed mental TLC. I hadn't seen Mahankirn since before surgery, and we spent the first ten minutes catching up. After our session, she said, "Wow. You are a haunted house inside."

Yup. She pressed into a couple of spots on my palm, which really hurt. She said the pain is from my *chakras* being blocked. (The seven main energy centers in the body—*chakras*—can become blocked from sickness, loss, anxiety, stress, and fear. Apparently you're supposed to keep them clear in order to achieve total balance in your mind, body, and spirit.) Mahankirn gently massaged my palm until the pain subsided and my whole body relaxed. She is magical.

Before I left we talked about my future. I'd been planning to look for a job as soon as chemo is done (September 15th), but she instructed me to take time to heal from this trauma. She suggested waiting until after Christmas to job hunt and said I should be kind to myself—get massages, go to the beach, sit outside, etc. In theory, I like the idea, but I'd have to drag around a puke bucket with me.

Maybe I could bedazzle a bucket, paint it pink, and stencil on some letters to say, "Kim Tronic's Fuck It Bucket."

_____

Friday, August 4, 2017

Chemo Session #12. This is the first time I've gone to a chemo treatment still feeling like shit from chemo the week before. Thank God there are only six sessions left.

Today I got Taxol in my tummy. I was irritated I couldn't move during the session, but it wasn't bad. The anti-nausea meds eased the weeklong sickness hovering over me. Was great to feel relief. I threw on my Mardi Gras outfit (beads, the Medusa green wig, gold mask), and I wanted to ask people to lift their shirts for beads, but somehow that felt improper in the chemo ward.

_____

Sunday, August 6, 2017

Post-Taxol days are easier than Post-Double-Dipper days. I'm struggling, but I'm slightly less of a disaster this weekend compared to last.

Last night Jon and I ate dinner at Mess Hall (appropriate, considering my mental state), and I couldn't finish my meal. We both got teary over how hard this has been. The smell of cheese almost made me puke. We wanted cocktails but decided against it.

This afternoon Jon and I went to Kara's. She was serving vodka lemonades, but we resisted. Not drinking is not fun. But we met a fantastic guy named Jeff who runs a nonprofit that helps homeless people around Los Angeles. Jeff is kind and sincere and probably the most grounded guy I've ever met.

I had a lovely conversation with Kara, who helped me realize I ought to get outside more. Being cooped up last week gave me cabin fever. I'm feeling a strong urge to camp, hike, sunbathe, and connect with nature. Kara invited me to go camping in November, and I can't wait! I'll need to invest in camping gear (not that I should spend money on extraneous activities, but fuck it) and cease watching scary movies about the woods. I hope we're not planning to camp where they filmed *Blair Witch Project*.

Tuesday, August 8, 2017

I finally had coffee today! The smell doesn't disgust me, which is an improvement. Coffee is my queasiness barometer.

Went for an hour-long walk and loved being outside. Definitely very out of shape. I got winded walking up a hill that I used to sprint up. But it's difficult to assess my health and fitness, because my weight keeps jumping all over the place. I was down to 145 (close to my goal weight!), but one day of chemo put me at 148, then a day of fluid put me up to 154, then a week later I'm at 152. I'm done trying to control it.

Wednesday, August 9, 2017

Dare I say that today is the first day I've felt not only OK, but actually *good*? Knocked out a two-mile treadmill run and morphed into bald Superwoman. I invited Celeste over for a dip in the pool. I met her at the same tech startup as blue-haired-Anne. Celeste is a crazy talented videographer who's got the cutest smile I've ever seen. I'm glad we're still homies even though we don't work together anymore, and I'm so proud of her. She's young (twenty-two, I think) and already has her life together. Sometimes I forget she's fourteen years younger because she's so mature.

Celeste came by and we splashed around in the pool for awhile, then grabbed dinner at (where else?) Hamburger Mary's. Our server was the adorable darling who served us when I had my "See Ya

Later, Ovulator!" cake a month ago. He remembered me and asked how I've been. I was honest about how much life has sucked, and he brought me a special sparkling water with lime and mint in a huge glass shaped like a leg, complete with a high heel and fishnet stockings.

Celeste is planning an international trip with a buddy and they're both buying a one-way ticket to Japan. How cool is that? They're gonna backpack around and see where they end up. Makes me want to travel. Life is short, and I clearly have no time to waste.

Thursday, August 10, 2017

Woke up queasy, which surprised me, since I felt great yesterday. Took a Zofran and ate some cereal. They should make a cereal called Zofrano's for cancer patients. The oats can be infused with metal, since that's what everything tastes like.

Kara and TK threw a party to celebrate their five-year wedding anniversary. It was on the rooftop of Mama Shelter, a cute boutique hotel in Hollywood with great views. Kara texted and said she wanted to do my makeup for the party, so I zipped over to her place at three. She brushed on layer upon layer of highlighter, bronzer, eyeshadow and everything else, including fake eyelashes. After an hour, I looked in the mirror and gasped. I'm not used to seeing myself with a heavily made up face. I *loved* it. I never knew how sexy fake eyelashes could be. Sure, it felt like a caterpillar was glued to each eye, but I looked gorgeous. Who says cancer can't be sexy?

I threw on my red wig (Alexis) and the beautiful polka dot dress that I bought the day before surgery. I felt fierce.

Jon and I had a blast at the party. We chatted with Jeff, the cool guy who runs that nonprofit, and drank a bunch of champagne. (Yeah, yeah, I know I *shouldn't* drink and put extra strain on my liver, but it's been a shitty summer and it's a special occasion, so don't fucking judge me, OK? Plus, I heard it's bad luck to toast people with water, and I can't handle any more bad luck.) Kara served a scrumptious homemade chocolate peanut butter cake, and Jon and I inhaled a couple of pieces then came home.

After taking off my dress, makeup, and wig, I looked like a hairless ogre once again, but at least I felt cute for a few hours.

Saturday, August 12, 2017

Was so nice not having chemo yesterday! The schedule for chemo is different now than it was before surgery. My first nine sessions were once a week, every Friday. Now they're two weeks in a row, then a week off. It's great having some extra time to recover.

Michelle came to visit today. She dated my brother Rob in college and it didn't work out, but she's always remained a part of my family. She lives up in San Francisco and drove down here to see me for a few days. She booked an Airbnb right down the street and got here around eight p.m. Jon and I took her to Sun Cafe for vegan food. I haven't seen her in forever, but catching up was easy and fluid. I'm awestruck by her. She has a terrific job working with diabetic folks (mostly children), but she's planning to go back to school and get a nursing degree. She does yoga, Pilates, and loves cats. She's kind of my soul mate.

During dinner I explained the whole situation to Michelle (which I now refer to as the official Cancer Journey Recap), and Jon's eyes welled up. I feel bad that he has to constantly hear this story over and over when I tell it to friends. I mean, he lived it—and we're still in the thick of it.

To lighten the mood, I told Michelle the story from a couple of weeks ago when I drank espresso and took cannabis oil and debated calling 911. The sad tears turned into happy laughing tears.

Sunday, August 13, 2017

Jon and I took Michelle to Venice Beach. We met TJ, one of my brother Rob's besties from high school, for lunch. I haven't seen him in probably twelve years. We had a great time—the food was tasty, the weather was perfect, and the reminiscing was gut-busting.

TJ and Michelle played around in the ocean while Jon and I worked on our (nonexistent) tans. We strolled along the boardwalk to peruse the funky art and jewelry, and TJ bought me a cool piece of the Los Angeles skyline.

After the beach, we grabbed a quick dinner and saw *The Big Sick*. It was hilarious, but some scenes hit too close to home. The main character's ex-girlfriend is in a medically-induced coma, and seeing her family at the hospital reminded me of getting diagnosed, surrounded by *my* family. I could tell those scenes affected Jon, too, because I saw him quietly wiping his eyes. We'd been sharing a huge popcorn, so our napkins were covered in oil and butter, and we had no choice but to smear buttery residue across our faces to wipe away the tears. We left the theater with swollen eyes and shiny salty faces.

I half-jokingly scolded Michelle for picking a movie that was too true to life. She felt awful, and during the drive home she meekly asked, "Wait, are you seriously mad?" Obviously I wasn't, but I appreciated that she's so neurotic she had to ask. I would have done the same thing.

Thursday, August 17, 2017

Jon and I decided to book a trip to Sedona for my birthday. I've heard the vortexes out there are supposedly very healing. According to VisitSedona.com, vortexes are "swirling centers of energy that are conducive to healing, meditation and self-exploration. These are places where the earth seems especially alive with energy. Many people feel inspired, recharged or uplifted after visiting a vortex." A little more hippy-dippy than my normal M.O., but my instincts tell me this is exactly what I need.

I did some research and scheduled a couple of excursions. Jon and I will arrive on Friday, September 1st, and stay in a beautiful hotel with stunning views of the red rocks. On Saturday (my birthday!) we have a vortex Reiki healing session, and Sunday we'll do a vortex *chakra* healing tour. Monday we'll check out and drive home. I'm so freakin' psyched for this. Originally Jon and I had been kicking around the idea of heading to Catalina for some birthday beach cocktails, but spiritual awakening sounds better.

Also, my final chemo treatment is less than a month away! I can't believe it. I remember thinking this horseshit would never end.

Friday, August 18, 2017

Chemo Session #13. Was very proud of today's chemo costume. Dressed as the devil. Horns, tail, large pitchfork, and red wig (Alexis). Several people, both nurses and patients, stopped by to compliment my ensemble. I like when people stop by. It feels like cocktail hour. Patients usually have some semblance of privacy, so we don't interact too often, but when I wear bright, crazy shit, it catches their eyes and they pop over. One elderly lady really made my day. She hobbled over, frail and pale, but had a huge smile.

"I love your outfit. That's so cute," she remarked. My heart melted. These costumes cheer other people up, which cheers me up.

I had only Taxol today, so treatment sailed by. Jon and I have been binge-watching *Silicon Valley* on Netflix, and it's wonderful. The writing and acting are flawless. And since I've worked at two start-ups, I can relate firsthand to the annoyances of digital tech. Every punchline on this show cracks me up. Jon and I plow through like nine episodes each time I have treatment. (Seriously, if you've never seen it, please do yourself a favor and check it out on HBO Go. The first season contains a situation that's referred to as the "best dick joke in TV history.")

Also, turkey sandwiches are dead to me.

Not looking forward to Cisplatin tomorrow. Next week is gonna suck.

Saturday, August 19, 2017

Chemo Session #14. Dressed like a pimp for treatment. Blue jean vest, gold teeth, a Pimp cup (a faux-diamond encrusted chalice, aka jewels glued to a plastic cup), and a fake roll of money. I felt cool. And I wanted to trick myself into thinking that I'm tough so maybe Cisplatin wouldn't be so terrible.

The nurse was super nice, but she didn't administer Ativan or Benadryl (which help me relax) with my pre-meds, so I felt flustered and treatment dragged by. I'm not sure why she didn't give me the Ativan or Benadryl. Maybe it was an honest mistake, or she thought I didn't need them. I should have said something, but I didn't. Adding to my agitation was the fact that I wasn't allowed to get out of bed because of my tummy IV. *Silicon Valley* was the only reason I kept my sanity. At least Sedona is only a couple of weeks away.

Tuesday, August 22, 2017

I'm flipping the fuck out. My kitty Riley threw up a few times, so Jon brought him to the vet while I was at Cedars getting fluid hydration yesterday. The vet said it could be his pancreas or thyroid, and today they called to say his blood work came back fine. Which means it could be something much worse, like cancer. This morning Riley wasn't eating or drinking, so we may have to keep him hospitalized while they figure out what's going on. This is the absolute last thing I can handle.

I'm so sick from the Cisplatin, and this kitty drama is making it worse. I felt like garbage all day. I was crying and queasy and it was pure hell. There's no way my cat can have cancer while I have cancer, right?

Life's not that unfair, is it? Is it?

Wednesday, August 23, 2017

The vet called and said Riley's stomach looks warped, so we had to bring him to another vet who can do an ultrasound. We rushed him to the new vet and waited while they did the ultrasound, which showed a mass in his stomach. The doctor said we should do surgery immediately, and we left the vet sobbing and praying. They won't know if the mass is cancerous or benign until the biopsy comes back, which will take a few days.

I'm a fucking *mess*.

Thursday, August 24, 2017

Thank God Riley's surgery went well. The kitty doctor said he removed the entire mass from Riley's intestine, and also removed one swollen lymph node. But we still don't know anything without the biopsy results.

I visited Riley at the vet, and he seemed OK. I felt super nauseated, but nothing was gonna stop me from seeing my baby. They put us in a small private room, and it was nice to pet him and watch him walk around. He seemed like his normal self. He crawled onto my lap and purred, and I told him he's a good boy through a steady stream of tears. Praying that he doesn't have The Big C.

Friday, August 25, 2017

Chemo Session #15. Tummy Taxol. I felt so queasy this morning, I couldn't bother to throw on a costume. Amazing that I'm this sick from last week's Cisplatin treatment.

I came dangerously close to puking all over my chemo bay. Even the anti-nausea meds barely helped. Then my stomach turned sour, and I wondered if I would make a mess in my pants. Cisplatin is the fucking devil.

I pouted for ten straight hours.

Have I mentioned I hate turkey sandwiches? And now I've started hating Honey Graham crackers, which used to be my Cedars comfort food. At least there are only three sessions left.

Saturday, August 26, 2017

Riley is back home, but he's wearing the awful "cone of shame" until his stitches come out, which is Tuesday, September 5th. The other cats are being rude and hiss at him. Breaks my heart. And Riley won't eat or use the litter box with the cone, so I have to take it off, then quickly put it back on. This is stressful.

Mildly queasy. Still waiting on Riley's biopsy results.

Monday, August 28, 2017

I decided to push the Sedona trip a few weeks. I don't want to leave Riley until I know what's going on, and heaven forbid something happens while I'm gone, like he pops his stitches or develops a complication from surgery. I would never forgive myself for not being here. So the trip is now scheduled for Friday, September 29th through Monday, October 2nd. Plus, chemo will be all finished by then, so we can truly celebrate while finding spiritual enlightenment.

Went to the DMV to renew my license. Refused to have a bald head in my license photograph, so I wore one of my expensive nice wigs (Vicka). I made the appointment weeks ago, so I got to bypass the hundreds (well, dozens) of people waiting in line.

I was nervous I wouldn't pass the vision test. I've become progressively more blind over the last few years, but I've been too lazy to get glasses. When I got to the guy's kiosk, he said to read the letters on a sign above his head, and I had butterflies in my belly. Then I had to cover one eye and read more letters. Shit. I could feel myself squinting, but I managed to squeak out the right answers. Then I covered the other eye and squinted so bad my whole face scrunched up.

Thankfully the man seemed to hate his job and didn't care about my vision. I zipped over to the photo kiosk and gave an uncomfortable smirk for my picture. I left fifteen minutes after I arrived. When did the DMV get so efficient?!

Wednesday, August 30, 2017

Panicking about Riley. Last night he vomited a *huge* amount. I thought his head would spin around. I called the specialty vet where he had his surgery, and they said puking once is normal, but if he does it again, bring him in immediately.

This morning he ate normally, but there was a weird orange-red puddle near the litter box. I rushed him to the vet but had to wait an hour since I was a walk-in. The tech took him back for vitals, an x-ray, and a urinalysis. While I was waiting, the surgeon guy said they finally had the biopsy results. It's cancer.

What. The. Actual. Fuck.

It's called Intestinal Adenocarcinoma. And it had spread to Riley's lymph node. The doctor recommended I bring Riley to see a kitty oncologist, who can discuss treatment with me—aka kitty chemo.

Apparently it's not as harsh as human chemo (shudder), but just the thought of Riley and chemo freaks me out.

The doc also said that even with chemo, I'll probably only have another year or two with Riley, at most. I cried so hard I couldn't breathe. Riley's only twelve. I won't be ready to say goodbye in a year or two! But without chemo, any microscopic cancer cells in Riley's body will likely metastasize, since it already did once. *This is bullshit.*

Jon came home from work, and we spent the evening weeping. Having to deal with cancer myself is one thing, but watching my sweet, helpless feline deal with this disease is just cruel.

Friday, September 1, 2017

Called the kitty oncologist and made an appointment for next week. I've heard good things about this doctor from a friend who also had a kitty cancer situation.

No chemo for me today, so Jon and I went shopping. First we hit the pot shop and talked with the owner Frank for a while. Frank is awesome. He sat with us for over half an hour, going over the benefits of cannabis oil for pets. He showed us three testimonials from people who have supposedly used Rick Simpson THC oil to cure cancer in their dogs. Dogs and cats can't be that different, right? The only thing I'm hesitant about is that Rick Simpson oil is super potent and makes you high. I don't want Riley to be stoned out of his mind. So Frank suggested we start Riley on CBD oil for a week (which is non-psychoactive so there's no high) and see how he does, then switch him to the Rick Simpson oil. I liked that plan, so we purchased the CBD oil, hugged Frank, and zipped over to Santa Monica.

We browsed around a couple of hippyish mystical stores. Jon bought a book about clearing and connecting with your *chakras*. I got candles and a couple of crystals. Both stores had calming music playing, and the energy felt spectacular.

Jon gave Riley his first dose of CBD oil. Understandably, Riley didn't like having liquid squirted into his mouth, but if it will help, I'm all for it.

Went to dinner with Jon and Ashley. We ate at The Dresden, and I had salmon for the first time in years. It definitely tastes different now. It used to taste like, well, fish, and now it tastes like fish that's been marinating in metal and loose change. *Damn you, taste buds.*

Ashley got a cocktail with serrano peppers, and I liked it so much I drank half of hers and ordered one of my own. Listen, before you scold me for drinking yet again, let me remind you I drank only a few times in the last five months, and that's a major accomplishment for me. I obviously want to keep my body as clean as possible, but cancer has taught me that life is short. Relax and have a fucking cocktail.

Saturday, September 2, 2017

Happy birthday to me! Turned thirty-seven today. Where did my thirties go?

Mom and Dad sent flowers, a balloon, and a ginormous fruit basket. Jon and I ate seventy percent of the fruit and immediately developed stomachaches. Jon gave me a princess balloon and beautiful red roses. We toyed with the idea of going to a comedy club, but lethargy prevailed, and we ordered pizza and watched *Ozark* on Netflix.

I've started burning sage every day, and it calms me. Maybe it's just the placebo effect, but I'm in a better mindset now.

Sunday, September 3, 2017

I've been thinking about my career (well, lack thereof) a lot. Maybe I should be open to a new kind of job. I mean, I love marketing, I love writing, I love the digital tech realm. But I was laid off from two startups in that space, so it might behoove me to consider something different. Especially because I'll need stable health insurance after this.

Something that really appeals to me is writing children's books and educational material. I began jotting down ideas for a kid's book, and it's so fun. I've been writing little poems and jingles since middle school, and it comes to me very naturally, but I never thought to explore this route. I'll need to give it more thought.

Riley sat on my lap twice today, so he's being more social. He's clearly feeling better, and that makes me feel better.

Tuesday, September 5, 2017

Took Riley to get his stitches looked at, and the surgeon said he looks great. Today he jumped up onto my bed for the first time in weeks. And he's not hiding under the bed all day like last week. I think I'll switch him over to the Rick Simpson THC oil after I meet with his oncologist.

Had a fantastic dinner at Mohawk Bend. Met up with Alice, this total sweetheart with whom I connected on Instagram. While I was in the hospital for surgery, she found my page and sent a message saying how I inspired her. We started texting all the time, and today was the first time we met face-to-face. She has cervical cancer and underwent a hysterectomy around the same time I did. Alice's treatment will be five straight weeks of radiation with a few chemo sessions peppered in between. She's bubbly, kind, and easygoing, and I loved having a buddy to relate to. I can't wait to see her again.

Nervous about tomorrow's appointment for Riley.

Thursday, September 7, 2017

Took Riley to the oncologist, and I felt terrible about stuffing him in his cat carrier for a long car ride. His doctor said that even with chemo, Riley will only have about a year left. Without chemo, he'll only have six months, and the cancer will spread.

Crying. This is so fucked up.

Riley's chemo treatments will be similar to mine—two weeks on, then one week off. Then we repeat that cycle three more times. Allegedly he won't have awful side effects—there shouldn't be any vomiting and very little appetite loss. Still, the thought of my baby with poison in his body breaks my heart. I decided to start his chemo today, so they gave him an injectable version during our appointment. He also got an ultrasound, so we could have a baseline to compare against his final ultrasound after the four cycles. Thankfully the doctor said she didn't see anything alarming, meaning no new growths or lesions in his lymph nodes.

I have to wait a couple of weeks to switch Riley to the Rick Simpson THC oil. I'll start on Week #3 when there's no chemo, so if he experiences any side effects, we'll know it's from the oil, and not the chemo.

Spent most of the day in tears. But at least Riley ate a lot when we got home, so he must feel decent. I can't muster that much excitement about my own chemo ending soon, because his just began. I feel like I'm starting all over again.

Is the Universe pranking me?

Stress-ate three cookies, half a bag of Skittles, and two cupcakes. Then remembered that cancer loves sugar. *Shit.*

Friday, September 8, 2017

Chemo Session #16! Wow. Just one week left. I can clearly remember the beginning of this path and thinking it'll never end. That I'd never make it through. That this entire year would be shrouded in a heavy cloud of shit. And it was, but at least my shit is almost done so I can focus on Riley's shit.

Since I had only Taxol in my arm IV, it was a quick day. Watched a few episodes of *Ozark* and snacked on a sandwich. My Angelic Nurse Practitioner Corina stopped by during treatment to see how I'm doing. I told her what Jon and I are planning for my final session next week—we're getting a cake with Dr. Li's photo scanned onto the frosting, along with a dozen cupcakes for each nurse station that spells out "We Love Cedars." Corina said Dr. Li will get a huge kick out of seeing his face on the cake. Doesn't everyone want to eat their own face?

Saturday, September 9, 2017

Chemo Session #17! *Finally* the last belly Cisplatin. Thank God. I slept OK last night but woke up at dawn and couldn't fall back asleep.

I thought today would suck, but my nurse was a total pro, and I didn't even feel the needle sliding into my belly. She was also super fast, and we were done in four hours. Previously the Cisplatin took around seven hours. So our nurse definitely had magical Nursey Powers. And knowing it was the final Cisplatin made it even better.

Started re-watching *Silicon Valley* on Netflix during treatment. And started hating all cookies from the nurse station. So now turkey sandwiches, Honey Graham crackers, peanut butter crackers, and oatmeal cookies are dead to me. I think any food my brain correlates with chemo will ultimately remain blacklisted forever.

Tuesday, September 12, 2017

Oh, hello, nausea, you wicked bitch. I bet you missed me. Nice to see you again.

For some reason, my pharmacy only gave me fifteen Zofran pills, when the prescription was for thirty. I called the pharmacy and they said my insurance would only cover half and I would have to wait another two weeks until they'd cover the remaining pills. Sorry, but WHO IS THE ASSHOLE AT THE INSURANCE COMPANY THAT HAS THE POWER TO DECIDE HOW MANY PILLS A CHEMO PATIENT SHOULD BE ALLOTTED EACH DAY?! This is some serious bullshit. I know that insurance is necessary, but what the fuck am I paying for if I can't get cancer medication?

FUCK YOU, BlueShield.

I have shooting pains throughout my whole body. Sucks, but good to know the Cisplatin is working its way through my system. It's the weirdest sensation. The tops of my feet, tops of my hands, ankles, and knees hurt the most.

I felt so sick on my way to get IV fluid hydration that I hung my head out the car window and wore a dark t-shirt in case I puked. I insisted on getting some anti-nausea meds along with hydration, and those eventually helped. It's SUCH a drag to be at the hospital five days in a row. Everything annoys me—especially the dripping and beeping noises from the IV machine. Those sounds grate my nerves over and over until I want to scream and rip the needle from my arm. Thank God this is the final week. I don't think I could make it through another cycle.

Thursday, September 14, 2017

Holy shitballs, tomorrow is my final chemo treatment! No more turkey sandwiches. No more Honey Graham crackers. No more dragging my IV chemo pump through the hallways to use the restroom. And no more poison in my body. I never thought this day would come.

Speaking of chemo, today was Riley's second treatment. Instead of a chemo shot like the previous appointment, this time the poison was in pill form. I had a pit in my stomach during the drive over—I

HATE that my furball has to go through what I went through. I tried to sneak the chemo pill in a Pill Pocket (little treats that have a built-in pocket where you hide medication), but the lil' bugger spit everything out after a couple of chomps. So the vet tech shot the pill down his throat and he took it like a champ. Thankfully his blood work came back normal and he seemed fine when we got home.

My post-chemo narcissism program is moving full steam ahead. Tomorrow I'll ask Rockstar Cancer Ninja Dr. Li when I can plan for Botox, Restylane, a new tattoo, laser spider vein removal, and buying a Corvette (OK, fine, maybe a Ferrari). It'll be nice to not cringe every time I look in the mirror.

Friday, September 15, 2017

Can someone please cue, "We Are The Champions" by Queen?

Chemo #18 baby! Final treatment day. It's so surreal.

Picked up the cake and cupcakes on my way to Cedars. The cake was legendary and turned out better than I anticipated. Dr. Li's photo looked great on the frosting, and the decorator snazzed up the design with fondant stars. The cupcakes smelled intoxicatingly delicious, and I knew the nurses would love them. I came dangerously close to eating one in the car.

Jon and I dropped off the cupcakes at both chemo wards and posed for a few photos with my favorite nurses. But the highlight was Dr. Li's reaction when I presented his cake. He dissolved into a fit of laughter and I could tell he was touched. I took a mental snapshot of the moment, savoring the love and euphoria in the room.

We composed ourselves, and Dr. Li congratulated me on reaching the finish line. I bombarded him with questions about nutrition, vaccines, follow up visits, and my prognosis. I'll come back in three weeks to remove my arm and stomach ports. Starting in December, I'll come back every three months for blood work and a pelvic exam.

He told me about Lynparza, a "remission pill" that we should consider. Apparently the FDA recently approved it, and studies indicate that BRCA-positive patients have responded really well. It could drastically increase my chances of staying in remission, but the side effects sound shitty. (Nausea and fatigue, just like chemo.) Dr. Li said we don't have to decide right now, but it's something to think about, and we can revisit the discussion in December.

I was hoping he would offer assurance that I'm forever cured, but he didn't. Even though I'm now in remission and statistically have the best odds of long-term survival, there's never a guarantee. I wished I had a better sense of security about my future, but I suppose cancer deprives you of that.

I started feeling super queasy as chemo began, but the anti-nausea drugs kicked in, and treatment went smoothly. A bunch of nurses came by and thanked me for the cupcakes. I got a lot of hugs, took a lot of pics, and told a lot of jokes. It was the perfect way to end treatment.

As Jon and I strolled toward the exit, I thought, *Wow, this is it. I'm done. This is my final trip down Chemo Street. I'm no longer a chemo patient—now I'm a fucking survivor. Where's Gloria Gaynor when I need her?*

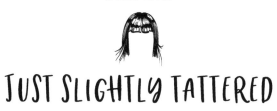

[PART FIVE]

JUST SLIGHTLY TATTERED

Saturday, September 16, 2017

I thought I would wake up and dance around my apartment. Throw a one-woman party. And scream from the rooftops that chemo is no longer on my To Do list.

But I didn't. I feel bummed. Sad. Stagnant.

My brain churned with a flowing current of doubts and fears. *Will I ever get married? Or adopt/purchase a kid? Own a house? Get a rescue dog? Why don't I have those things now?* It's frustrating to see people my age (or younger) checking off these life milestones, while I've checked off none. But why am I stressing about this now? I should rejoice today, and focus on what I *do* have. Perhaps I should stay off Instagram so I won't spiral.

Went for a walk with Jon to clear my head, and the warmth felt good on my skin. Jon suggested we hit Umami because he knows Impossible Burgers always cheer me up. (If you've never had one, bookmark this page, leave your house immediately, and go get one.) They're legitimately the best, most realistic veggie burger in the world. Apparently they're made from wheat, coconut oil, potatoes, and heme (which is an "iron-containing molecule that occurs naturally in every single plant and animal," according to Impossible's website). They taste like meat. They feel like meat. They even "bleed" like meat. They're incredible. They're delicious. They're Impossible.

(This is not a paid advertisement for Impossible—I just really like the burger, OK?)

Monday, September 18, 2017

Saw Mahankirn (my energy healer) today, and OMG was it helpful. She made a great analogy—she said basically I just endured a giant tornado, and even though the turmoil has passed, I'm still standing among the rubble and devastation. It will take several months to pick up the pieces and recover. She could tell my nervous system is a wreck. After the session, the tension in my back was gone, and I felt serene. I didn't even get road rage on the drive home.

With a sudden urge to prepare a healthy dinner, I pulled into the Whole Foods parking lot and immediately realized my mistake. There were about fifteen cars circling the parking lot like vultures, desperately looking for a spot. I sullenly waited in a line of cars just to leave. How are there so many people wanting to buy overpriced food at two p.m. on a Monday? Doesn't anybody have a job? Sheesh. I popped into Ralph's, where parking was aplenty.

As I surveyed their wild-caught salmon, a woman with a gorgeous baby strolled up beside me. The woman also examined the fish selection, and the baby and I met eyes. I smiled at the baby. She tilted her teeny head, then slowly opened her mouth and started to scream. *Geez, kid, am I that scary-looking? Or can you just sense my desperation for a baby?*

I Googled "How To Cook Salmon" and followed the recipe. Shockingly, the fish turned out perfect. I was surprised I didn't mess up. And more surprised I actually felt like cooking. That energy healer really knows what she's doing. Maybe she can teach me how to wear high heels, too.

Wednesday, September 20, 2017

Woke up with fresh resolve to find a job. Scoped out some interesting opportunities in L.A. and applied for a writing gig at a box subscription company. Just for shits and giggles, I also checked out listings in Boston. I applied for a writing job at SharkNinja, because I love their vacuums and blenders. I'm not sure I'm ready to move to Boston at this exact moment, but I figured it can't hurt to expand my search to both coasts. I hate the idea of leaving Jon and palm trees and friends and sunshine behind—my entire life is here—but I'm filled with an intense longing to be with my family, and it's overriding everything else.

Tried a smidge of the Rick Simpson THC oil for the first time. The dose was so tiny I didn't feel stoned. Tomorrow I'll try a little more. I'm determined to wean off Temazepam (for my chemo-induced insomnia) because I don't want to depend on prescription meds for sleep anymore. Sadly, I was wide awake from three to six a.m., but I productively used that time to analyze everything that's gone wrong in my life and count the number of stains on my wall. I also thought of some very clever comebacks for arguments that I had with people eight years ago.

Thursday, September 21, 2017

Took Riley in for blood work this afternoon to make sure his body is handling everything OK. Thankfully, he didn't need chemo. His levels came back perfectly normal and the vet tech said it seems like he's doing well. Whew, maybe he and I can have a Remission Party together!

Applied for another writing job in Boston, this one for a company that makes educational materials. I'd never seen myself working in education, but now that I want to write children's books and videos, I'm open to new career trajectories. I may even open myself up to selling fruit on the street corner or joining a Ponzi scheme.

I felt like cooking again (seriously, did hell freeze over?!), and I found these awesome veggie patties made from pea protein, called Beyond Beef. Cooked those up with olive oil, salt, pepper, garlic, and cayenne. I'm very proud. I mean, I realize that some people cook for themselves every day, but this whole thing is new to me, so can we please just give me a round of applause for not blowing up my kitchen? Thanks.

Friday, September 22, 2017

Boston, here I come! Booked a nine-day trip, from Saturday October 14th to Monday October 23rd. I can't wait to chill with my parents and see my niece and nephew and brothers and jog around my quiet hometown. Everything feels safe there. It's the antithesis of how I feel in L.A.—like danger lurks around every corner. Going to the beach? Hope you enjoy tsunamis. Cruising down Sunset Strip? Prepare to get T-boned by some asshole on his phone. Taking a nice hike? Watch out for earthquakes and brush fires. At my parent's house, there are no threats of natural disasters. And cancer can't follow me there. (My cancer ran out of frequent flier miles, so it doesn't travel.)

The Sedona trip is one week away. Getting really psyched for the Reiki and *chakra* healings, and hoping I can leave my anxiety behind in L.A.—along with the toothbrush I'll inevitably forget.

Cammy called and asked if I wanted to hang. Cammy's the greatest—she always seems to know when I need something, and we clicked the moment we met. She'd been wearing an adorable houndstooth jacket, and I kept joking I would steal it, and voila— our friendship was born. Unfortunately, she's a jerk and donated the jacket a few years later instead of giving it to me. Anyway, she invited me to a cool musical showcase for veterans that our friend Michelle was attending. The vets spent a couple of hours creating a song about their combat experiences, then performed it onstage. The song was touching and beautiful. One girl cried as she sang, which made everyone in the audience cry. After the performance, we all had snacks and chatted. I could feel a nice sense of camaraderie among the veterans and it got me thinking—maybe I should seek out a cancer survivor community. It's reassuring to speak with people who have a deep understanding of your pain and fears, and who also survived the same hell you endured.

After the event, Cammy, Michelle, and I grabbed some Mexican food. I figured I deserved a splurge since it was my first official post-chemo weekend. I had two (OK, three) jalapeno margaritas and 200 pounds of chips and salsa. I only ate a few bites of my chicken fajitas, because my stomach was about to explode from all the junk I'd just stuffed into it. I'm so gonna regret this tomorrow, but it was worth it.

Saturday, September 23, 2017

It wasn't worth it. I slept like crap, probably because my body was like, *Excuse me, what did you just do?* My face is hilariously bloated and I now have a double chin.

Jon and I went to see *IT* and I enjoyed it. I'd never seen the original series, but I liked the adaptation. Of course, I had to have popcorn with the movie. And now the theater allows you to bring in cocktails from the lobby bar, so I splurged again. (OK, OK, I know, I know…alcohol may increase my risk for a recurrence. But am I supposed to *never* drink again? Fuck that. I deserve to live a little, and everything in moderation.) My face is gonna be so gross tomorrow. I'm anticipating three chins and a whole lotta face flab.

Sunday, September 24, 2017

Yep, three chins now.

Time to get back on track and eat healthy. Cancer loves junk food. *What the fuck am I doing?!* I'm in remission, and I need to stay that way. I will *not* let those shitty tumors grow back.

My sweet Instagram buddy Alice is having a tough time with the side effects from chemo and radiation, so today I brought her cannabis oils and edibles. I can't understand why her doctor won't give her a cannabis prescription, especially considering that recreational marijuana will be legal here in a few months. It's silly. She shouldn't have to suffer with these side effects when cannabis would so easily help her. Stupid red tape bullshit.

I've been taking the Rick Simpson THC oil the last few nights, and I still haven't experienced a high, but I'm starting to sleep better. I took ZzzQuil last night and got a solid seven hours of slumber. And really, beauty sleep has never been so important, considering I look like a decrepit ogre. Honestly, there's no amount of sleep that will make me feel attractive at this point. I've thought about rubbing butter all over my mirrors so I won't have to accidentally catch my reflection while brushing my teeth.

Tuesday, September 26, 2017

Last night I decided not to take any sleeping pills and nodded off for only three hours. This whole "weaning off pills" thing will take a bit more finessing. There are few things more frustrating than staring at the ceiling at four o'clock in the morning, but I did get a chance to count the stains on a different wall, so that's good. I also thought of more witty comebacks to arguments circa 2005.

Looks like the family is taking a cruise for our holiday vacation. I'm so freakin' happy we'll all be together. Kicking back poolside.

Throwing back cocktails. Celebrating the end of a shitty year. Even though I'm morally and ethically opposed to cruises because of their environmental impact, I'm thrilled the whole clan will have some fun together. But I'm a little apprehensive about my health—I've heard cruises are a cesspool for germs. Didn't we all hear that news story about a norovirus outbreak which made hundreds of people sick? Gross. And I don't have a spleen, so I'm extra susceptible to bugs. I should head to Costco for a 400-gallon drum of antibacterial hand sanitizer. But I'll finally get to swim in the ocean for my post-cancer victory vacation.

Really want a damn job soon. I applied for another opportunity in Boston and another in L.A. Now it's up to fate to decide my...fate.

The last few nights I've been sly about giving Riley the Rick Simpson THC oil. I snuck it in Pill Pockets and treats. But the other night, he refused to eat anything, so I smudged a few dots onto his tongue. He immediately started drooling and foaming at the mouth. It was scary. I was like, *Oh God, did I overdose my cat?!* Eventually the drooling slowed down, but he hid under the bed for the rest of the night, and I felt like the worst pet parent on earth. Tonight I tried to revert to the Pill Pocket and treats (and even tried turkey and cheese), but the oil is so pungent he can smell my trickery from a mile away. I want to scream at him and make him understand this will help him. Irritating.

I'm still astounded that my cat and I concurrently got cancer.

Thursday, September 28, 2017

Brought Riley to the vet for a chemo injection, which kicks off Cycle #2 for him. Poor little bugger. He threw up as soon as we got home. The kitty oncologist said he looks great, and even gained a bit of weight. Now we're at week four of twelve, so we're almost halfway there. I just hope he will accept the THC oil in his nighttime snack moving forward.

Popped into the grocery store for water, popcorn, bananas, and granola bars for the Sedona trip. I hate long car rides (this one will be seven hours), but it's better than flying. Some comedy CDs and good music should make the drive somewhat tolerable.

Next week I'm getting fake eyebrows! I'd never heard of microblading before this, but now I'm obsessed. It's semi-permanent cosmetic tattooing that looks so real, you can't tell it's not actual hair. Cammy referred me to this awesome girl in Valencia, so I made an appointment. My face looks weird without bangs or eyebrows or eyelashes. This situation truly helped me grasp the importance of facial hair (excluding peach beards, obviously). I just want to slap the girls who overpluck their eyebrows and be like, *DO YOU EVEN KNOW HOW GOOD YOU HAVE IT?* Never again will I take hair for granted. Shit, at this point, I'd even settle for a mustache. Which may not be so off the radar, thanks to menopause, and at least if that happens, I can easily update my name from Kim Tronic to Jim Tronic.

Friday, September 29, 2017 | L.A. TO SEDONA

I forgot how much I hate road trips. Well, I don't hate the entire trip, just the part where I'm stuck in the car for hours and hours and hours. I get bored, and I need to be entertained at all times. Sitting in the passenger's seat for seven hours is a huge challenge for me. I wish I were one of those people who can put their feet on the dashboard, read a book, and enjoy the long stretch of road, but I get carsick easily, and I'm too fidgety.

We stopped at a couple of Starbucks along the way and listened to a million comedy CDs. I was cranky and felt trapped inside our metal box for most of the journey. But then...the cacti and red rocks came into view and *BAM!* Instant excitement. Also, instant congestion. My nose got stuffy and I kept sneezing. Am I allergic to Sedona? Let's hope not.

As Jon and I navigated the entrance of Enchantment Resort, we were stunned by its beauty and seclusion. We checked in and a dude named Reilly (like my cat!) drove us to our room in a golf cart. Actually, the room was technically a *casita*, which means we had a separate kitchen with a fridge, microwave, stove, table, and cabinets full of plates and cutlery. The incredible living room had a fireplace, a bed that folded into the wall, and a super comfortable couch. And the balcony...the view was unreal. We had a total 360 view of the red rocks. A sense of peace washed over us. *Finally.*

We bellied up to a bar at the resort's restaurant for dinner, and the food was exquisite. My salad was colorful, fresh, and delish. I had a cactus plum margarita, which sounds gross, but it was so light and sweet, I sucked it down in four sips. While we ate, the lady next to me chatted us up, and we had an awesome conversation. Her name is Laura, and she'd lived in Sedona for thirteen years. I started to wonder what it would be like to live here. It's got a small town vibe, which means I would miss the exciting nightlife of a city (aka, have the freedom to order takeout at midnight), but the slower pace of life seems awfully appealing right now.

After dinner we walked back to the room ('scuse me, to the *casita*), but our key didn't work. So we scurried back to the lobby and they reprogrammed the key. We went back to our *casita* but the key still didn't work. *What the fuck?* We went back to the lobby again, and they seemed to think we were going back to the wrong *casita*. We hitched a ride with one of the resort employees...and they were right. Jon and I were trying to get into the wrong *casita*. But in our defense, the *casitas* were set up so that our room, 137, was in between rooms 237 and 337. *Not* in numerical order. How does that make sense?

Jon and I smoked a CBD joint on our balcony, and I focused on the lack of noise. The only sounds were crickets and a crisp breeze. And we could see the stars in the sky, a luxury not afforded to us in Los Angeles. After the weed, we cuddled on the couch and watched

Fuller House on Netflix, and I raided the mini fridge for thirty dollar gummy bears and a fifty dollar bottle of wine. (Sure, I *should* have snacked on the crushed granola bars in my purse, but cancer gave me a sense of entitlement, so I felt I earned some obnoxiously over-priced candy and booze.)

Saturday, September 30, 2017 | SEDONA

Slept terribly. Jon and I jolted awake at one a.m. to creepy noises coming from the walls and roof. Ghost? Raccoon? Who knows. We were freaked out and wide awake for a couple of hours. I finally conked out around five a.m. then got back up at seven. Despite the lack of slumber, I enjoyed the morning and snapped some solid Instagram pics from our balcony.

We ate breakfast at Mii Amo, Enchantment's sister resort that was a quick five-minute walk across the property. Toward the exit of Mii Amo, we noticed this little circular nook off the lobby called The Crystal Grotto. The floor was covered in red sand, and a small waterfall surrounded the crystals in the middle of the room. I noticed a slight vibrating sensation in the air, and my feet tingled. Jon and I sat silently in there for a few minutes, and we each shed some tears. I think we both wanted so badly to release the buildup of sorrow from the last five months, and this was the place to do it. We ran into Reilly during the walk back to our *casita*, and he said that the grotto was built on the edge of a vortex, so it's no surprise I felt tingly.

Jon and I didn't know what to expect from our Reiki On The Rocks excursion, and we went into it with very open minds. Our tour guide, Chris, picked us up and asked what we hoped to achieve in today's outing. I delved into my official Cancer Journey Recap, which I'd perfected by now. *It was a dark and stormy night, and I had pains in my upper abdomen...*

Chris drove us to a vortex, and we began our hike, stopping to take in the scenery a few times. I felt like I'd been transported into a beautiful painting, surrounded by deep shades of red, green, and blue. A childlike giddiness grew inside me, and I kicked at pebbles as we ascended the mountain. It was impossible not to smile.

We found a nice ledge toward the top and sat down. Chris spritzed us with his homemade smudge spray (which smelled so good I later purchased a bottle) and instructed us to do breathing exercises. My feet tingled again. I tried to hone in on my senses—the sounds of the birds, the tickle of the breeze, and the warmth of the sun. Cancer was the last thing on my mind.

We meditated for a few minutes, then Chris led us to a nearby park. He spread out a comfy blanket and told me to lie down and close my eyes while he did Reiki. (Basically healing me through the art of touch by channeling energy into me.) I felt a calmness that I hadn't experienced in a long time. *Everything will be OK. Your hair will grow back. You'll stay in remission. Riley will be ok. I don't know why Chris is fanning me with bird feathers, but it's fine.*

Back at the resort, I noticed how tired and congested I was. Could that be all the emotional toxins leaving my body after today's nirvana? We smoked a post-dinner CBD joint and binge-watched more *Fuller House* before tucking into bed.

Sunday, October 1, 2017 | SEDONA

Slept a little better and woke up at seven. Gulped down two heavenly cups of coffee and waited outside for today's tour guide, Jared. He picked us up, and I gave him the Cancer Journey Recap on the way to Bell Rock, one of Sedona's most powerful vortexes.

Somehow, today's view was even better than yesterday's. We did a few yoga poses, and Jon and I kept toppling over, because we're not very balanced—mentally or physically. We moved on to a guided meditation, and Jared told us to envision ourselves on a beach, with ocean waves gently lapping over our legs.

In that moment, I immersed myself in the sights and sounds of my environment—the soft breeze, the sun on my skin, and the lovely birds chirping, and it hit me—*OH. This is what it means to be present in the moment. No worries. No anxiety. Not a care in the world. Nothing but that which surrounds me. This is what true freedom feels like.* It was similar to what I felt during Reiki yesterday, but this level of tranquility went a lot deeper. I felt unattached from the omnipresent uneasiness in my soul—at least for a moment.

Jared took us to another vortex, and we talked about the power of fear. I told him about the anxieties that constantly plague my mind: politics, cancer, finances, unmet goals, the veins on my legs, the size of my ass. He pointed out that all of these worries are rooted in fear. You can't let fear dictate your life. All you have to do is break down the barriers that fear has created. Hmmm. I'll need to ponder that after I have a sandwich.

As we drove back to Enchantment, I contemplated that crazy moment of fulfillment from today's meditation. Jared wanted me to understand that if I felt that way today, I can feel that way all the time. The ability is inside me, and I can tap into it anytime I want. *Whaaat? Would that even be possible in Los Angeles? Possible in the apartment where I spent all those months on the couch, sick, unemployed, and miserable? Possible when I'm stuck in traffic and want to bash my head against the windshield? Possible when I'm watching all the bills pile up and looking at my negative bank balance?*

Monday, October 2, 2017 | SEDONA TO L.A.

Noooooo. I don't want to go home. I need to stay here for another week. Or forever.

Jon and I set the alarm for seven a.m., inhaled some coffee, and hiked up Boynton Canyon, the vortex next to our resort. We climbed as high as we could and squeezed in one final meditation. The breeze seemed full of positive energy and we shed ~~a few~~ lots of tears. It was the proper way to cap off our trip.

We grabbed smoothies at Mii Amo and reluctantly packed our suitcases. We weren't quite ready to leave Sedona, so we stopped at The Secret Garden Cafe for lunch. Our cute patio table overlooked a garden (duh), and each table had a blanket to keep its customers warm. I ordered a water, a cappuccino, and a Bloody Mary so I could cover all my basic beverage groups. Our server totally understood my infatuation with this town. She'd initially visited Sedona in 2007, then later came back for a few days, then later for a week, then finally moved here for good. I made a mental note to do the same.

Jon and I meandered into a cool store next door and bought some books, candles, sage spray, and a small bottle of red rock sand (that way I could bring a little piece of the magic home with me). As I paid for my bounty and struck up a conversation with the cashier, a woman overheard us and approached me. She introduced herself as Liz, and said my story resonated with her, and she could feel my positive energy. Liz asked for a hug and we embraced for a moment. *Was I emanating good vibes already?*

The journey home wasn't bad. The mountains and cacti faded into the background, and I silently reflected on the mystical weekend. I definitely felt happier, healthier, and better equipped to deal with all the shit waiting for me back in L.A. With only a couple of hours left in our drive, I threw on some great '80s tunes and clutched the bottle of sand. I examined the teeny red particles and thought, *Maybe Jared is right. Maybe, just maybe, the magic is inside me.*

Wednesday, October 4, 2017

I miss Sedona. Now that my body is physically recovering, I need to continue the mental healing as well. I'm still sort of Zen, but I can feel my road rage creeping back in.

Had a phone consult with this alternative healer lady, per the recommendation of a buddy. Apparently she analyzes your blood and recommends supplements based on her findings. My buddy said she really helped him when he had health drama, so I agreed to talk to her. I had sent her a drop of my blood in the mail (sounds creepy, no?) and written down a sample of what I eat on a daily basis. Oh, boy, was she full of shit. She told me I have a parasite, as well as high levels of arsenic and yeast. Best part? The "cure" for my parasite is to go on an eight-day food fast and drink nothing but goat's milk. I don't think it takes a genius to figure out that denying my body of food and nutrients and vitamins is the exact *opposite* of what I should be doing while I recover from chemo. And she had the cojones to charge 800 dollars for the phone consult, blood analysis, and a bunch of her company's branded supplements. Go fuck yourself, lady. Those bottles of snake oil went directly into my recycling bin.

Sunday, October 8, 2017

Kara hosted Sunday Funday, and the food was *delish*. I'm getting psyched to camp with her next month. But I'll need to make a conscientious decision not to fret about serial killers lurking around our campground. Does that only happen in the movies? Or do serial killers actually hang out in the woods with their guns and machetes and flannel shirts, just waiting for unsuspecting idiots like me to come visit?

I walked back from Kara's, my heart full of love and laughter, but things plummeted when I got home and logged onto Facebook. I flipped through photos on Jared's page (the tour guide from Sedona) and I felt pangs of envy that he's married with four beautiful kids. *Why can't I have the things I want? A house, a dog, a marriage. Cancer has forced me to seriously evaluate what I want in life, and now I truly understand time is the most precious commodity. How long am I supposed to wait to go after what I want?* I love Jon so much, but these frustrations, which have bumped around in my mind for a while, now reside at the forefront of my brain. I have no time to waste. I do want to marry Jon, but I know he's not ready at the moment, and it kills me. I looked at Jared's photos and sobbed and let myself wallow in self-pity for the rest of the night. It was pathetic.

Thursday, October 12, 2017

Got my arm port removed today!

It was a surreal mind-fuck to sit in that waiting room. Back in April, I fidgeted in the same chair, nervously awaiting my first day of chemo. Today I came back victorious, excited, and eager. The waiting room looked exactly the same, but I had a totally different outlook.

The doctor who extracted my port was the same one who'd installed it. But this time I actually welcomed his presence, and we jammed to classic rock during the procedure. Amazing to think how far I've come in six months. After he stitched me up, I got to see the little passport that resided in my arm, and it was *bizarre*. This small rubbery triangular contraption was responsible for sucking up the chemo drugs through an IV and dispensing that shit throughout my body. Weird how such a teeny, innocuous object can wield so much power. I was struck by the amount of relief that rushed through me, as if the excision became a physical representation of the cancer and suffering getting pulled out of me.

Now that chemo's over, Jon is playing more gigs, which makes him happy, which in turn makes *me* happy. I felt guilty that he put everything on hold for me. Music is a huge part of his life, and I'm glad he can do what he loves again. The way he feels about music is the way I feel about writing. We've both got a creative outlet where we're free to express ourselves. Except he's super talented, and much of what I write is verbal diarrhea.

Friday, October 13, 2017

Today marked the final milestone before we officially move from Kill Cancer Mode into Surveillance Mode—I got my tummy port removed!

I loved seeing Rockstar Cancer Ninja Dr. Li in a setting that didn't involve chemo—this was a triumphant occasion. Just like yesterday, I was totally awake and lucid during the procedure. They numbed my stomach area around the port, and Jon stayed to watch from across the room.

We all joked around while Dr. Li swiftly prepared. As he injected the numbing medicine, he said, "Here comes a little prick," and Jon and I simultaneously replied, "But he's sitting in the chair." *Zing*.

I told Dr. Li about the quack healer who said I should go on a goat's milk cleanse, and he shook his head and had a sour expression on his face. *My thoughts exactly*. Dr. Li said I need all the healthy food I can get, and depriving myself of proper nutrition would be foolish. Doing that "cleanse" would not only slow my recovery, but potentially set me back and introduce new complications. The American Cancer Society recommends at least two to three cups of fruits and veggies every day, along with healthy fats, lean proteins, and healthy carbs to ensure you get the necessary nutrients and vitamins for recovery. And I'm much more inclined to believe Dr. Li and the American Cancer Society than some "doctor" who charges hundreds of dollars for her own supplements.

I packed for Boston and realized that baldness equates to a lot of extra room in my suitcase. No hairdryer, shampoo, conditioner, flat iron, or self-esteem.

Saturday, October 14, 2017 | L.A. TO BOSTON

Man, I detest flying. All morning I was terrified about bad turbulence. At one point, the plane started bumping around, and I
grabbed my teddy bear from my backpack and clutched it until the
turbulence ended. That's right, I'm a thirty-seven-year-old woman
and I still have a teddy bear.

Mom and Dad picked me up at Logan Airport. We chatted about
everything during the drive home (*Yes, I feel OK…Yes, I still hate being
bald…Yes, my anxiety is awful…Yes, Jon is hanging in there…No, I don't
have any job prospects…Yes, I do feel skinny but I'd rather be slightly fatter
and not have to worry about cancer …*), then stopped for coffee because
I needed a hazelnut Dunkin' Donuts.

Cancer feels so far away right now. It's like a game of hide-and-
seek. It can't find me at the moment, but I know it's out there, hunting me down.

Sunday, October 15, 2017 | BOSTON

I love waking up here. Those first few moments where you emerge
into lucidity are peaceful and soft, unlike waking up in Hollywood,
where you're forcibly shoved into consciousness from shrieking car
horns, people shouting, and cop car sirens.

Went for a run with Mom, and we knocked out four miles. The
scenery was majestic, and everything you'd expect from a New England autumn: colorful leaves, crisp air, and chirping birdies.

Rob and Vasanti (my brother and his wife) brought the kids over
for dinner. They're so big! Anika is talking now. Weird. She's an actual human. I'm so infatuated with her. She runs around from room
to room, but her legs are unstable, and it's like watching a baby
gazelle find its footing.

Kiran gave me a huge hug, and all the love melted me. I'd bought
the kids some very cool bracelets in Sedona (remember those "slap

bracelets" from the '90s?) and they seemed to adore their fun new wrist wear.

Kiran gave me flowers he'd picked himself, and it blew my mind. My brother hadn't even suggested Kiran get me flowers—my little homie had the idea all by himself. Kids can be so thoughtful when they're not yelling, breaking things, or making a sticky mess. It warms my heart to see how happy my parents are with their grandchildren. It all reinforces that eventually I wanna adopt a baby girl. I've even picked out her name already. Veronica Tronic. And, as quoted by Homer Simpson, "Kids are great. You can teach them to hate the things you hate." Fantasized about cancelling my flight back to the west coast and staying here forever.

Tuesday, October 17, 2017 | BOSTON

Saw Tina (my BFF from high school) last night. She was in North Andover visiting her mom for a couple of days, so I popped over, and the three of us hung out. Her mom is having a rough time. She's been battling cancer ever since I've known her, and it's metastasized to her brain. She's hanging in there, but you can see treatment has taken a toll. My heart breaks for her and Tina. We traded war stories, and despite the somber mood, we laughed about our shared baldness, and I busted out my favorite cancer joke. (I pull the wig cap—which looks like pantyhose—on the top of my head and exclaim, "Cancer patient!," then pull it all the way over my face and exclaim, "Bank robber!") Tina and I went out to grab some takeout, then we all ate together. I headed back to Mom and Dad's with a full stomach and heavy heart. God, cancer is such a cruel, shitty disease.

Mom and Dad took me to Joe Fish for dinner tonight. I ordered a five-pound lobster and felt bad about eating it (*sorry, little guy*), but it tasted scrumptious and felt very New England of me. I vowed to return to vegetarianism at some point. I wore my bright red wig (Alexis) and felt people staring, which caught me off guard. In L.A. no one notices piercings, wild outfits, or bizarre haircuts. But people in this small, quaint Massachusetts town aren't accustomed to seeing anything out of the ordinary.

Toto, we're definitely not in Hollywood anymore.

Wednesday, October 18, 2017 | BOSTON

OK, as much as I enjoy quiet suburbia, the lack of city background noise exacerbates my tinnitus. During the day, I don't notice the tinnitus, but without white noise at night, the ringing in my ears drives me nuts.

Weighed in at 144 this morning. Holla. Usually I gain weight when I come home, but this time I'm eating tons of veggies and avoiding the snack closet I normally dig into.

I drove to Boston for a visit with Abby (a bestie from college). She's got two gorgeous little sons with huge personalities and bright blue eyes. We decided to check out the local playground so the kiddos could monkey around. Jamaica Plain (Abby's beautifully diverse neighborhood) seems like a lovely place to raise a family. Watching all the little tykes running around, I felt a pang of envy and knew if I had ovaries, they'd pulsate with a desire to start my own family. I probably looked liked a creeper, staring at the children with a wistful expression on my face. Thankfully, no one called the cops to report me.

Enjoyed a spectacular homemade dinner with Mom and Dad. Had a great conversation with Dad about his job in pathology, gratitude, and life in general. He's more cynical than I am, but he acknowledges we're lucky to have a kickass family. Dad agreed with my sentiment that the most important stuff in life is the intangible stuff—love, friendship, and family.

Friday, October 20, 2017 | BOSTON

OMG. Sore throat galore. I forced down a coffee because #caffeineaddiction, but I probably should have had tea. It hurts to swallow. Sat around watching movies all day. Weighed in at 145 and I feel fat.

I'm really needing (and wanting) a job. I'm approximately two weeks away from selling everything I own to a sketchy Hollywood pawn shop. I have to publicly apologize to my bank account, because it's embarrassed to be associated with me. I mean, the unemployment checks are still rolling in, but it's barely enough to get by. I know I'll get back on my feet in 2018, but I'm anxious for a steady stream of income, not a sputtering trickle.

Jon called and said Riley's chemo went well today. The kitty oncologist thinks Riley looks great and continues to maintain a healthy weight.

Sunday, October 22, 2017 | BOSTON

Dug around online for job and apartment listings in Boston. Got depressed. The affordable apartments were tiny with bad carpeting. The job posts were a joke—$40K a year for a Marketing Manager? Wow. How does anyone afford a house around here? I need to reevaluate my career choices.

Got lunch with Mike (my ex-boyfriend from college). He picked me up and we drove to New Hampshire. I can't believe he's married now. And sells insurance. He's sure changed from the wild stoner I used to know. I hadn't seen him in over a year, and we talked about marriage, cancer, kids, etc.

I told him about my crazy journey and said I'm considering adoption since I'm now *sans uterus*.

He said he'd NEVER adopt a kid—adopted kids tend to have

serious mental and emotional problems, and he'd rather have no kids than adopt one. He then proceeded to tell me about his cousin who adopted a girl from Korea, and had to spend thousands of dollars on therapy for her since she's so maladjusted.

Super helpful, Mike. Thank you. It's not a sensitive topic or anything. Asshole. You were a lot nicer when you took bong hits and wasted your dad's tuition money on cheap beer.

Felt bummed the rest of the day, but put on a happy face. Sore throat kicked in again before bed, but wonder if that was my resentment toward Mike bubbling to the surface.

Tuesday, October 24, 2017 | BOSTON

Still heated about Mike's adoption rant, but I know I need to let it go. Those are his issues, not mine, and carrying around that animosity will only drag me down

Did a mountain of laundry and started packing. Rob brought the kiddies over for dinner, and I savored every moment of family time. Anika's little wobbly run melts my heart. One day I want to tell her she was single-handedly responsible for eradicating my hatred of children. I also had a good time holding Kiran upside down. I hope they think I'm a cool auntie.

Wednesday, October 25, 2017 | BOSTON TO L.A.

My flight back to L.A. was smooth, but my seat neighbor kept coughing and sniffling and wiping his nose on his sleeve. I heard him tell the girl on his other side he'd gotten sick a few days ago. Normally I'm not a germophobe, but I have no spleen and a compromised immune system, and I could practically feel his dirty germs burglarizing my body. I tried to breathe in the opposite direction and vowed to swallow a bottle of antibacterial gel when I get to Hollywood.

Had a pleasant Lyft ride home, and the cats were desperate for my attention as they clamored for a spot on my lap. Tomorrow I'm gonna take Riley to the vet, then see Dave about getting the rest of my arm tattooed. This was the tattoo I was *supposed to* get on the, "Good morning, you have cancer" day. At long last, I'll have my inky redemption—a literal way of etching cancer's conclusion on my body. *Take that, tumors!*

PART SIX

KEEP CALM AND KIMMY ON

Thursday, October 26, 2017

Dear jet lag, I loathe you. Love, Kim.

I'm still on east coast time. Woke up at six and could not fall back asleep. I miss my family already.

Today Riley was due for a chemo pill, which marks the end of Cycle #3—just one more cycle to go! It's literally impossible to administer the pill myself (have you ever tried shoving a pill down an angry cat's throat?), so I brought him to MASH, the specialty vet that did his surgery. They got him to swallow the medication and I gave him a fistful of treats. How come no one fed me treats during my chemo sessions?

Went to see Dave Parker about my tattoo. The top part of my sleeve will have a sun, ocean waves, and an outline of Massachusetts. Masshole for life, baby! (For non-Massachusetts residents, Urban Dictionary defines a Masshole as "an obnoxious loudmouth who takes pride in his aggressive and illegal driving habits. They are too cool to use turn signals. Massholes say things like 'wicked' and 'pissah' and 'go fahk yahself, kiddd.'")

After dinner, Jon and I went to Kara's Halloween party and had a blast knocking back a few (too many) vodka/sparkling waters.

Once we got home, Jon and I plunged into a long drunk emotional conversation, the type where you say all the shit that's been festering in your gut but don't feel comfortable sharing without a boost of courage from Lady Liquor.

It ripped a hole in my heart. He feels like I don't support him. That I never really thanked him for taking care of me during cancer. And basically, if I move to Boston, I'm making him choose between Los Angeles and me. I realized I never thought about things from his perspective. I just want to be near my family and return to a place that I love. But now I understand the situation as he sees it—that he'd have to move across the country and give up his life in L.A. to be with me. I smoked a CBD joint to shut off my brain, but it didn't work. It made me want ice cream.

God, I've been a selfish bitch. How did I not recognize this?

Friday, October 27, 2017

OK, it's time to start seeing a therapist.

I'd been mulling it over for months, but I never got around to it—partially because I was embarrassed, and partially because I wasn't sure if I really needed to. I've tried to stay strong throughout the turmoil, and I thought asking for help would make me weak. Maybe I wanted to prove to myself that I'm a tough cookie. But I'm so overwhelmed with questions and fear and doubt that therapy feels like the only solution.

Spent hours hunting online for local psychologists. Eventually I found a therapist network and I submitted the digital form to request an appointment. Got a call from their office later in the day saying, Sorry, all the psychologists are completely booked and not accepting new patients. I got fucking waitlisted. Is everyone in L.A. so messed up there aren't enough shrinks? It's not like I'm trying to buy a limited edition Louis Vuitton purse for heaven's sake—I just need someone to talk to.

Jon and I stayed in and got takeout. I told him I felt shitty about last night's convo and apologized for not thinking about things from his perspective. He understood, and we made peace over pad thai. I'm grateful we have amazing communication—it's a huge reason why we've had such a long-lasting relationship.

Saturday, October 28, 2017

I told Mom and Dad I wanna start therapy. I was SO nervous to share the news, but I'm not sure why. I knew they wouldn't judge me, but maybe I was afraid that my bubbly, tough-as-nails exterior would look a little tarnished. To my delight and surprise, Mom exclaimed, "That's a great idea!" I'm sure my neighbors heard my heavy sigh of relief.

Went to a kickass Halloween party at Hadley's. I dressed up as a devil, using the same costume that I wore to Kara's on Thursday, and Jon went as a sparkly angel (appropriate, considering what a saint he is). He looked good with glitter all over his face. I brought vodka and flavored sparkling water, my new favorite cocktail.

Spent a little time in Hadley's room giving love to his kitties. If I'm ever at a party and there are cats or dogs, I immediately cease all human interaction and smother the animals with kisses for the duration of the evening. I also made some amazing cancer jokes ("Hey, Taylor, can you grab me a vodka? I have cancer!"), but I'm not sure everyone thought my quips were funny. People don't seem to know if it's OK to laugh, which I understand, but laughter is like the *only* thing that helps me heal.

Sunday, October 29, 2017

Jon and I watched the season finale of *Ray Donovan*. I love that show, but it was terribly difficult to watch some of the scenes where his wife was dying of cancer. I'm glad my prognosis is great, but seeing her pale skin and weak body is like a painful flashback. *That was me, just a few months ago.* I know eventually it'll get easier to face those types of visuals, but my emotional wounds are still too raw and tender right now.

Thinking I should step up my search for a full-time gig. I need to work. Having this much spare time is wearing on my nerves. Even the cats are tired of having me around every day. And I'm starting to hate my living room. The furniture feels old and dull. The color scheme bugs me. Even the view outside my window pisses me off. *Is it normal to resent a bookshelf this much?*

I'd been debating whether I should mention cancer in my job interviews, and I concluded I won't. I'm not ashamed—I just don't want a potential employer to look at me differently. I want them to consider me based on my skills and writing portfolio, not on sympathy or empathy. I also don't want them to think, *Oh, maybe she'll need time off for doctor appointments.* Or maybe I'm just projecting my insecurities and should stop overanalyzing everything. Perhaps this will be something to tackle in therapy.

Wednesday, November 1, 2017

I spent an hour at Jetrag looking for something fun to wear to Kara's Busted Barbie comedy show on Friday. I found some cute corsets that were either way too small or way too big, which made me feel too fat and too skinny. Then I went home and suffered a meltdown in the bath. Those awful hair follicle bumps have returned, and this time they brought their friends. They're everywhere. On my neck. On my back. On my shoulders. On my legs. I sobbed.

This is bullshit. I no longer have disease in my body, yet cancer still finds a way to fuck with my vanity and psyche.

I did some research and discovered a lot of women seem to have this problem after finishing chemo, and the bumps should disappear after a few months. Oh good, I won't look hideous for much longer. Or maybe I can paint my skin gold and just pretend those grotesque black bumps are cheetah spots.

Thursday, November 2, 2017

I'm trying to forget about the "follicle debacle" and focus on things I CAN control. Today I zipped to Valencia for an eyebrow touch up, and despite the numbing cream, it was agony. But my eyebrows are amazing and my face looks more normal. And my eyelashes are getting longer! My face is like a half-finished jigsaw puzzle—needs more work, but it's coming together.

I found a therapist! He's a super sweet guy named Bill I met a few years ago at a USC/UCLA mixer. I remembered his website, so I submitted a request form, and we had a fifteen-minute phone consult. He specializes in anxiety, depression, and career counseling, which is perfect because the things I need help with are anxiety, neuroses, and job shit. We'll have our first session next week, and I'm looking forward to it. Maybe I can finally get my head together. I don't know what to expect, but I bet it will go something like this:

Me: So, doc, thanks for seeing me.

Therapist: No problem, Kim. Let's start with why you're here today.

Me: Sure. I had ovarian cancer, I'm so full of anxiety that I feel like my heart is going to explode, I have such a bad temper that I break things, sometimes I binge eat, I'm scared of dying, I have no career, I'm terrified of North Korea, I'm uncertain about the future of my relationship, I cry all the time, my ass is huge, my skin is a mess, and basically I see myself as a sick, bald loser.

Therapist: <pushing button on intercom> Carol, please cancel the rest of my appointments this afternoon.

Friday, November 3, 2017

Loving my new eyebrows. I can almost look in the mirror and not recoil at my reflection. I kept glancing at my eyebrows in the rearview while driving to the laser vein removal appointment, and almost rear-ended a Hyundai.

I was wrong when I thought that the microblading was painful. Today's vein removal gave new meaning to the word "pain." The technician asked if I had a high pain tolerance, and I scoffed and showed her my tattoos. "Great!" she said, then handed me some goggles to protect my eyes from the laser. She made marks all over my legs with a pencil, then directed her little laser gun at each individual vein and began zapping

The first couple of zaps were pretty mild, like a hardcore bee sting, but it was tolerable.

"That's it? This is easy," I remarked.

Then...*BAM. ZAP. BURN.* FUCK. The pain was so intense I squealed. And squealed again. And again. The next thirty minutes were a mix of me yelling, apologizing, squirming, and wondering if this was worth it.

I whimpered the whole way home, legs throbbing, and got ready for Kara's Busted Barbie comedy show. I debated whether to wear a wig, but my head stubble is growing, so I resolved to be brave and rock the buzzcut. The breeze of the club's air conditioning on my head made me feel exposed and self-conscious, so I drank a couple of vodkas. I know it's only been about six weeks since I finished chemo, but it's hard to shake the lingering roots of cancer's attack on your ego. Alcohol definitely helps.

Sunday, November 5, 2017

Jon and I realized that we have virtually no camping gear, so we better get our asses in order, because we're leaving on Friday to sleep in the woods. We hit a sporting goods store and spent lots of money (thanks, credit card!) on pants and warm tops—apparently it's thirty degrees at night where we're going. Topped off the purchases with some sleeping bags, a tent, and two chairs from Amazon. I think we should be fine now.

Weighed myself, and now I'm at 147. Not terrible. I'll be happy if I can stay under 150, but it'll take a lot of self-discipline. Considering how scared I am of bears and axe murderers, maybe I'll be running a lot next weekend when we're in the woods.

Monday, November 6, 2017

Today restored my faith in humanity.

Cammy and I ate salads at Bossa Nova and chatted about cancer, therapy, our relationships, futures, and fears. The restaurant was packed, and our tiny two-top was close to another two-top occupied by a girl eating solo. I was trying to be cognizant of my speaking volume because I'm exceedingly loud. The girl was eating *caprese*, one of my favorite appetizers, and I tried not to stare at her food too much. Eventually she finished and left.

Cammy and I took our time, savoring tea and coffee after our food. When we asked to pay the bill, our server told us the girl at the next table paid for our meal and left a note that said, "Fight like a girl! XOXOXO." Holy moly. Immediately Cammy and I started happy-crying. We were blown away by this stranger's kindness and generosity. I couldn't believe a stranger would do something so selfless.

Our server said this girl is a regular, so Cammy and I asked our server to give her a note next time she comes back. We jotted down a sweet little thank you, and I instructed her to find me on Facebook. I hope she does. I would love to get to know this person. Anyone who makes a gesture like that is clearly someone who has a heart of gold, and is someone I want to know. And it made me think—shouldn't we all do things like that? Why can't we all look out for one another and be more altruistic? Isn't one of the main purposes in life to give back? Plus, if you're focused on other people, you're less wrapped up in your own bullshit.

Tuesday, November 7, 2017

Had my very first therapy session!

I adore Bill. He's warm and compassionate. Since it was our first appointment, we didn't dive deep into any one topic, but he explained a few key points. TFA stands for Thoughts, Feelings, Actions. Thoughts turn into Feelings which turn into Actions. So when I'm freaking out about stuff (*Will the cancer come back? Why am I not married? Why don't I have a house or rescue dog or savings account?*) that will turn into feelings (fear, anger, resentment) which turns into actions (panic attacks, running down the road screaming).

Bill also said that since my brain is constantly going, going, going, I need to get control of my thoughts, like I'm a conductor and my thoughts are the symphony. I dig that analogy because I always feel like I'm *part* of the symphony, in the middle of the loud noises and surrounded by the chaos and madness. But no, I can be *in charge* of that and be the leader.

We briefly touched on career stuff, and Bill said he believes that career opportunities seek us out, not the other way around, and I hope he's right. I think he will definitely be able to improve my mental health.

I've been sleeping better. For a while I'd wake up every night at three a.m., but the cannabis oils seem to help. I remember the Cedars nurses telling me that the insomnia and memory issues caused by chemo will take months to diminish, but I'm hoping I'm heading in the right direction.

Thursday, November 9, 2017

I took Riley to the vet for his chemo injection, which means just one more treatment then he's DONE! It was superhero day at the vet, and they had a photographer taking pics to celebrate the kitties and pups who are kicking cancer's ass. They had a cute little step and repeat in the lobby. When it was my turn, my doctor and vet techs wanted to be in my photo, because they were impressed that I beat cancer, and now Riley is (hopefully) beating cancer. It was a sweet moment and the pic is adorable.

I'm so ready for camping tomorrow. I probably over packed, but I hate when I'm traveling and end up wishing I had more socks or t-shirts or undies. I hit the store and got apples, bananas, granola bars, vodka, water, sparkling water, almond butter, cashews, and coconut milk. Kumbaya, y'all!

Friday, November 10—Sunday, November 12, 2017 | LOS ANGELES FOREST

I woke up early to get coffee and breakfast before hitting the road. I squished all my new camping gear into the trunk, picked up Bryan, and grabbed Eugene. We stopped at Sprout's for lunch and bought wine and snacks, because you can never have too much food or alcohol.

Once we got off the freeway and entered the mountain-y portion of the drive, I drove like five miles an hour. Those winding roads were terrifying, and I was sure we'd veer off the side and fall to our death, so I drove like an old lady. I didn't want to be inconsiderate, so I pulled over every twenty feet to let cars pass. It should have taken an hour to get there, but with my driving, it took about an hour and forty minutes. Thankfully, Bryan and Eugene were cool about it. *God, will there ever be a time when I'm not scared of EVERYTHING?*

We were the first ones at the campsite, so we unpacked and smoked a CBD joint. Our camping area was open and beautiful, surrounded by mountains, millions of trees, and a rockin' fire pit. I was happy about the flushing toilets because I refuse to use the forest as a restroom.

Jon and everyone else started arriving soon after, and they cracked open wine and champagne. It got dark early, around five. With no phones or TV or iPads, your perception of time gets really warped. We ate dinner (nachos and chili) and huddled by the fire to keep warm. Everyone dangled their feet over the fire pit, and four people ended up scorching their shoes. Burning rubber is a bad smell, but one that'll always remind me of this camping trip. Jeff brought hot chocolate and peppermint schnapps, which is now my new favorite cocktail for sub-forty-degree temperatures. I stupidly added a couple of vodkas to the mix and took a Xanax to help me sleep. It helped *too* well, and I passed out around two in the morning. Rumor has it I snored like a buzzsaw. In hindsight, mixing Xanax with alcohol wasn't the brightest decision, but at least I stayed unconscious and didn't worry about axe murderers.

Oh, fuck. I'm about to puke. Where am I? Why is my head spinning?

I woke up Saturday feeling like death. I got up to use the bathroom, then crawled back into my tent and napped until noon. I finally emerged and snacked on fruit and forced down water. The boys played horseshoe as the girls chatted. A bunch of us decided to hike up the mountain, and we got bloody welts and scratches from the surrounding shrubbery.

The view from the top was spectacular. I paused to take in the warm sun and strong breeze. It teleported me back to Sedona, when I felt totally at peace. I need more of these Zen moments. Maybe I can tap into this mindset more often by unplugging from technology, getting outside, and disconnecting from the anarchy in my brain.

OK, fine, I'll consider cutting down on my rampant Facebook stalking.

Back at the campfire, Kara and I talked about running. She asked if I'd ever want to run a marathon. I told her I'd already run four, and they kinda suck.

"Dude. We should do the one in L.A. in March! I've never done one, and we'd have a blast training."

I thought for a moment. I dug her enthusiasm, but was I ready to train for a fucking marathon? After my last one, I swore I'd never do another. And with the beatdown my body just endured, could it handle running all those miles? But then again, doing shit outside your comfort zone helps you grow, right? And this definitely counts—there's absolutely nothing comfortable about dragging your body along the road for twenty-six miles.

"Ah, screw it. I'm in," I replied, instantly regretting the decision.

Dinner was a burger bar and leftover chili. It was warmer than yesterday, so no one burned their shoes. I refrained from Xanax and booze and knew I'd sleep terribly. Everyone went to bed around eight, except Jon, Jeff, and I. We listened to music (and people snoring in their tents) and shared horror stories about coworkers.

Jon and I crawled into our tent at one a.m., and he promptly fell asleep. I lay awake, resenting him and everyone else for being able to nod off so easily. I'm an annoyingly light sleeper and need all conditions to be perfect to get good rest. At home, my pillows have to be perfectly arranged, my sheets have to be clean, my fan has to be on the right setting, I have to lie on my stomach, and my right leg has to be bent at a ninety degree angle. So, stuffing myself into a sleeping bag in the dead silent woods amidst an orchestra of mouth-breathers = the antithesis of an ideal sleeping environment. I angrily listened to the rhythmic snoring from my neighboring tents for about thirty minutes before I said fuck it, lugged my sleeping bag to my car, and curled up in the backseat.

Have you ever tried sleeping in the backseat of a Toyota Corolla? There's not a lot of space. I couldn't get comfortable. But at least it was quiet. Eventually I passed out, but I had a nightmare that some-one was standing outside the car and staring at me. *OH MY GOD, IT'S THE AXE MURDERER!* I woke up in a panic, on the verge of a heart attack. The axe murderer was actually a huge tree outside the passenger window. I lay awake for hours, glaring at the tree to make sure it didn't transform into a lumberjack.

Woke up to the sound of voices around eight a.m., and we all had coffee and broke down our tents. Jon drove my car back home, and those awful curvy roads had me queasy and worried that my cats would starve to death once the car plummeted off the side.

Wait, did I really commit to running a marathon next year? Crap.

Tuesday, November 14, 2017

Weighed in at 147. I still feel fat.

Dad wanted to talk to Rockstar Cancer Ninja Dr. Li about Lyn-parza, that "remission" medication. As a doctor, Dad insisted on get-ting the full report from an expert. Apparently they hopped on a call and Dad filled me in.

Lynparza sounds promising: studies have shown that it's effective in treating BRCA-positive patients who beat ovarian cancer then got a recurrence. But the side effects give me pause. Nausea. Exhaus-tion. And maybe leukemia. (Yeah, allegedly that's worst-case-scenar-io, but WTF? You can get cancer from a medication that's supposed to treat cancer?) I'll get more info from Dr. Li when I see him for my three-month checkup in a few weeks.

Kara and I went for a run, and yes, we really are doing the mar-athon next year. We had some great quality girl-chat, then talked about potato chips and cupcakes and steak and cheese, because all we do is think about food when we exercise.

Afterwards, I zipped to Studio City for a Botox appointment. I hadn't seen Lillith, my Botox Master, since last year, so I gave her the Cancer Journey Recap. She said I looked fantastic, and talked me out of getting fillers (injections that fill in facial wrinkles and give you a smoother appearance). Lillith recommended we only do Botox, and if I want fillers after the holidays, I can come back. That way my body would have more time to recover from chemo.

I wish I weren't so wrapped up in my appearance. It's aggravating to constantly fixate on the outside, when I know the real work needs to be done on the inside.

Thursday, November 16, 2017

Two great cancer milestones today:

1) Riley's final chemo treatment. I took him to the vet, and he handled it like a champ. I gave him treats and extra food, because everyone deserves a celebration when they finish chemo. Now I can quit "wishin' for his remission"—he's a healthy kitty.

2) Dave Parker inked on my amazing new tattoo. The design he put together is beautiful and elegant, and my upper sleeve flows seamlessly into my lower. It didn't hurt too bad...until he got to my elbow area. It hurt almost as bad as the laser vein removal. I'm sure Dave could see me grimacing through the pain. But after the pain of chemo and surgery, I welcomed this type of pain—a visual representation of the months of torment, and ultimately, the biggest victory of my life.

Monday, November 20, 2017

Spent an hour and a half on the phone with my health insurance. I keep getting bills from Cedars, even though I've paid my $4,000 out-of-pocket maximum, so I had to wait on the phone while my insurance rep sorted through that mess. Boring and irritating. The last thing I want to deal with after dealing with cancer is bills from dealing with cancer.

Did a sprint workout on the treadmill, but then I got dizzy and lightheaded, and had to sit down for several minutes. *Am I dehydrated? Or something more sinister? Could I have a cancer recurrence this soon? Or am I just out of shape? God, this shit is like PTSD.*

Met Bill for another therapy session. Why didn't I start this years ago? I told him how I feel kind of lost in terms of my career, and I'm tired of this omnipresent sense of uncertainty. And how I think everything I do is shit. Even blogging, which I used to love, seems like a chore, and I'm questioning my ability as a writer. *Do I really have what it takes to make a living at this? If I don't even like my own work, why would other people like it?*

In the miraculous way that he does, Bill shifted my perspective. He pointed out how terribly I speak to myself. I blamed cancer for breaking me down, but he said I'm not someone who's broken, who needs X, Y, and Z to be whole, to be a fully-formed person—I'm already complete. Hmm, I don't feel complete, but he was so confident, I believed him.

Damn, therapy should be mandatory for everyone.

Tuesday, November 28, 2017

I've gained about five pounds.

Yesterday I snacked on Thanksgiving leftovers all afternoon. The creamy mac & cheese tasted orgasmic and I was powerless against its rich buttery goodness. And if I'm being totally honest, I enjoyed the comfort that came with a reckless binge. But today I feel guilty.

Had another therapy sesh with Bill, and this time Jon joined us. I'm grateful Jon is willing to work on things together, and I didn't have to drag him there—all I had to do was bribe him with coffee.

It was nice chatting about our fears in a safe and nurturing environment with a neutral third-party referee. Every time Jon and I attempt to have these talks on our own, we get too emotional and cry and nothing gets resolved and I shut down. At least today, we could discuss everything and make some progress. We only got through a portion of what I wanted to talk about, so we're all going to meet again as a group next week. I think Jon and I both left the appointment feeling hopeful.

Last night Kara and I went for a jog with her friend Lisa. I'd only met Lisa once and I dug her sassy, bold, New Yorker attitude. I found out she'd battled cancer as well, and we had a very deep, honest conversation about our journeys. It's SO reassuring to hear other survivors' stories, and while I hate having a membership to the Cancer Club, I love knowing other people triumphed over the same anguish.

Lisa thinks I should be more vocal about my experience. Aside from keeping a diary and writing a couple of blog posts, I haven't made much effort to get my story out there. I guess I'm not sure how to go about it, but I like the idea of helping other people. Maybe they could find solace in my story, the way I found it in Lisa's—that'd be a cool way to flip the script.

Friday, December 1, 2017

Went to the weed store to get CBD oil, but there was a note taped on the door saying that they'd moved to a new location super far away. I got the urge to stress-eat, but instead of grabbing some calorie-dense junk food, I picked up eight bags of overpriced kale chips. I was proud that I made a healthy choice, but who spends eighty dollars on kale chips?! An unemployed cancer survivor, that's who.

Jon and I grabbed dinner at La Poubelle, and we had a great time. He applied for a new job, a couple of rungs above his current position, and felt good about his chances. I loved seeing him so chipper. His energy and mood were airy. His eyes sparkled. His face lit up.

We cracked a lot of jokes, and it felt like old times, before we ever felt the weight of cancer on our souls.

Saturday, December 2, 2017

Had a super scary dream about earthquakes and buildings collapsing and the apocalypse. I woke up terrified. I'd been stressing about the despicable GOP tax reform, which kind of feels like the death of democracy, so the dream makes sense. Stress-ate two bags of kale chips.

Jon had band practice, so I got takeout and chilled with the cats. He came by later and, for some reason, I thought it was a good idea to watch *The Belko Experiment*, a good-but-scary thriller about coworkers who are trapped in a building and kill each other. My anxiety skyrocketed. Perhaps I should refrain from films where murder is the main plot point. Maybe I should only fill my psyche with happy, fluffy thoughts like unicorns and puppies and glitter and pizza. I couldn't sleep. Kept tossing and turning. I listened to three different meditations before finally conking out around three a.m.

Damn you, Greg McLean. (*Belko*'s director.)

Tuesday, December 5, 2017

I've been thinking a lot about what Lisa said, and I decided to publish a blog post about chemotherapy. Eventually I'll want to share my story on a bigger scale, but this felt like a good start.

People responded well to it. The post got way more traction than my previous content, and I'm glad it struck a chord with everyone. I liked opening up, and I'll definitely continue to do so.

Went to therapy with Jon again. This time we tackled super dense topics like marriage, children, financial stability, and expectations in our relationship. It's so hard talking about that stuff, especially because we're not on the same page about a few things.

We went through a lot of Kleenex.

Bill wanted to know how we receive love from each other. Jon said he feels loved when I cook him meals, which I've started to do more often. *Huh, so the old adage is true—the way to a man's heart is through his stomach. Good to know.* I said I feel loved when Jon does things for me that are difficult for him, like coming to therapy.

I think we made decent headway, and I was relieved to express myself in a way that I'd never felt safe to. I'm certain Jon felt the same.

Went to a weed shop for CBD oil. They had a huge variety of CBD products, so I stocked up on edibles, joints, and bottles of oil. That "rollercoaster" sensation in my stomach is constantly happening, so my anxiety is worsening, but I hope the CBD can help. And really, what's there to stress about, other than cancer, Trump, the corruption in our government, my dwindling savings account, the pain in my tooth, my gray hair, my fat ass, and global warming?

Wednesday, December 6, 2017

Went to Cedars for a breast MRI.

I'd never had one, and up until today, I didn't know I was claustrophobic. But I stupidly had three cups of coffee before the appointment, so I felt super jittery. I had to lie face down on the platform, and as I moved into the MRI tube, my arms were squished into my sides, and I started to PANIC. I squeezed the little ball in my hand to signal to the nurse and screamed, "Let me out, let me out, let me out!"

She backed the platform out of the tube and I pulled off the headphones, nearly hyperventilating. I apologized and told her I needed a minute. She assured me it happens all the time. I took a few deep breaths and we tried again.

This time I focused on breathing and tried my hardest to relax. But my brain wouldn't stop rolling around in bad thoughts. Like, what if there were a fire alarm or terrorist, and my nurse had to run out of the building and left me trapped in this machine? What if the machine breaks and cuts me in half? It's totally feasible—something like that happened in those *Final Destination* movies. Or what if there's still some small amount of chemo in my body, and it reacts poorly with the contrast coming through my arm IV, and I melt from the inside out?

After a half hour, the MRI was over, and I gleefully skipped back to my car. I deserved a reward for making it out alive, so I treated myself to a new dress and fifty-dollar sushi platter.

Made a mental note to avoid coffee and get Valium for the next MRI.

Friday, December 8, 2017

The MRI results got posted in my Cedars Sinai app, and I freaked out at the word "cyst." *OHMYFUCKINGGOD, DO I HAVE BREAST CANCER NOW?!* The Breast Whisperer Dr. Dang said the cyst is benign. I sent the info to my dad, and he emailed back with, "The report is GREAT NEWS! RELAX! You do not have breast cancer and do not have any abnormality that is associated with increased risk of getting breast cancer. Breast cysts are common and utterly benign. A cyst (and yours is tiny, they said) is a simple cavity containing some fluid." Whew.

Zipped back to Cedars, this time for my first official "Post-Cancer-Three-Month-Checkup" with Rockstar Cancer Ninja Dr. Li. I can't believe it's already been about three months since my last chemo sesh. Time flies when you're ~~having fun~~ in remission.

I brought three trays of cookies, one for the short-term chemo ward, one for the long-term chemo ward, and one for Dr. Li.

I got to see a couple of my favorite nurses, Angela and Casey. It was rewarding and powerful to hug them now that I've crossed the finish line. I got teary-eyed. Those nurses are absolute heroes.

Seeing Dr. Li was equally sentimental. Now I could actually savor his company, instead of bracing myself for any potential bad news. He said I looked amazing and he patted my head. (I LOVE when people do that, so I probably giggled like a schoolgirl.)

I asked about that Lynparza medication, since he'd discussed it with my dad awhile back. Apparently, no, I wouldn't go on it, as Dr. Li discovered that it's FDA approved for BRCA ovarian cancer survivors, but only ones who had a recurrence. Since I'm in remission, it's not for me. So I won't take it unless the cancer comes back, but that won't happen. (*Right, God? Right? You wouldn't do that to me, would you? No? OK, cool, thanks!*)

I told him how I wanted to give back to Cedars in some way, whether through writing or speaking to someone or whatever, because I'd had such an incredible experience. Dr. Li said maybe I could talk to women who are about to go through what I went through.

Hell yeah, that'd be awesome! We hugged goodbye and I got a flu shot and quick blood draw to check my CA-125. We'll get the result on Monday.

Saturday, December 9, 2017

Jon and I went to my friend Babette's for dinner. I hadn't seen her or her husband Erik since last year, so we had lots to catch up about. Erik was one of my Marketing professors from UCLA, and I've been lucky to do a few freelance collaborations with Babette. I love that they're both entrepreneurs, they enjoy good food, good cocktails, and having lots of animals—perfect for me.

As we ate, I gave them the Cancer Journey Recap. By now, I've recounted this tale so many times that it's automatic—ten to fifteen minutes of summarizing my 2017 shit storm. Jon still gets a little upset every time I rehash the experience. But it's getting easier for me. I almost feel removed from the ordeal. The emotional beating I endured doesn't feel as fresh. Maybe I'm starting to believe that ultimately, I'll be OK—or I've just become desensitized to the story.

Sunday, December 10, 2017

T-minus only a few weeks 'til the holiday cruise! I checked out the website to see what kinds of activities are available on the ship (see also: what kinds of trouble I can get into). Aside from the typical vacation mumbo-jumbo (bars, restaurants, more bars, and a gym), there's a rock climbing wall, robot-staffed cocktail spot, casino, arcade, club, and rollerskating area. Cool!

The cruise ship departs from New Jersey, so my family and I will meet there. The boat will be at sea for one day, then dock in Florida for an afternoon. (No doubt my niece and nephew will wanna hit Disneyworld.) The following two days we'll dock in the Bahamas, at Nassau and CocoCay. Then the ship is back at sea for two days and docks back in Jersey. Ahoy, matey!

I'm psyched to drink a cocktail made by a robot. And to kick back, toast my family, and count my blessings that the worst year of my life is behind me.

Monday, December 11, 2017

Today rocked. Got two amazing phone calls from Cedars.

1. My blood work from Friday came in. A normal person's CA-125 tumor marker will be between one and thirty. Since I'm high-risk, they want me to stay under twenty. And last time we checked (in September), mine was five. So today I was hoping for ten or fifteen. But it's five! Great news. That

means my marker stayed exactly the same since I finished chemo. What a freakin' relief. *Good job, body!*

2. Sarah from the Cedars Community Relations Department wanted to discuss my submission for Giving Tuesday. Cedars launched a campaign inviting people to donate or share their stories of gratitude, so I sent them a quick paragraph about my experience. Sarah said my story made her cry (*hey, that makes two of us!*) and asked if she could feature it in their marketing collateral. Hell yeah! We'd do a photoshoot in January and set up an in-person interview. I immediately agreed. Sarah also told me about a potential writing gig on one of their content teams. If they move forward on filling the position, she wants me to apply.

Hey, maybe this is how I can give back to Cedars! AND get paid for it! Hello, dream job.

Tuesday, December 12, 2017

Went to therapy for another group session. Today was a million percent less draining than last time, but I learned a great lesson.

Bill had given us a homework assignment—take ten minutes to peel and eat an orange, then take ten minutes to write about it.

Jon nailed it, describing the orange's smell, taste, and texture. I completely fucked up, only focusing on the dialogue in my head like, *This orange tastes good, but why is my therapist having me do this assignment? Is he trying to get some grand realization out of me through this stupid fruit?*

I answered my own question. Instead of living in the moment, engaging my senses around the orange (like Jon did), and appreciating the details, all I did was worry about what Bill would think.

Well played, Bill.

After the orange discussion, we did a wonderful guided meditation.

The tension in my body melted away and my mind quieted down. I need to make sure I'm more consistent about meditation—some nights I'm too lazy or not in the mood. But since my body is healing, so too should my mind.

Tuesday, December 19, 2017

Ugh, why hasn't Cedars called with a job offer? I'd like to think I'm their biggest cheerleader…and I'm dying to get back to work and resume normal life.

Kara and I went for a jog, then she swung by, and we registered for the marathon. It's nonrefundable, so there's no backing out now. We decided we should probably loosely follow some type of training program. Godspeed. I didn't die from cancer, but I'm afraid the marathon might kill me.

Had a great chat with Bill at therapy today, talking about fearlessness versus recklessness. Like many people, I was fearless in my teens and twenties, thinking I'd live forever and nothing could hurt me. In fact, I used to be so fearless I was also reckless, making stupid decisions with no regard for the consequences. But once my thirties and cancer rolled into the equation, I became afraid of everything, which is a huge source of my anxiety.

After what I've endured, is it possible to not live a fear-based existence? Apparently, yes. Bill pointed out that running the marathon allows me to regain control and do things outside my comfort zone. And if I let fear dictate my actions, I'll never do anything significant or risky or great. That's great food for thought. *Oooh, food.*

Monday, December 25, 2017

Spent my very first Christmas in Los Angeles. (Normally I fly back east to see my family.) It feels weird and wrong not to have the

Tronics together, but I'll see them next week during the cruise.

L.A. is quiet. There's no traffic, and it's surreal. Jon and I went out for dinner, and I threw on a huge Santa hat and strung Christmas lights around my neck. The restaurant had a warm buzz of happiness, and people complimented my necklace. Jon and I indulged in a decadent meal and chocolate mousse for dessert. Back at home, we polished off a couple of champagne bottles and watched *Garfield's Christmas Special*, a very grainy holiday cartoon that my family and I have watched every single year since 1984.

Ugh, with all the calories I consumed today, it's a very Merry Bloat-mas, indeed.

Thursday, December 28, 2017

I met with a dermatologist for the first time ever. Last month, when I made the appointment, my skin was covered in those pesky post-chemo black bumps, but they've mostly cleared up by now. But I figured I should get my moles examined to make sure there's no skin cancer lurking in the shadows.

Thankfully, everything was fine. She said chemo tends to age your skin, and she could see the sun damage on my face. These sun spots across my cheeks wouldn't have been visible for another twenty years, but the chemo drugs pulled the sun damage to my skin's surface. Awesome. Fortunately that's fixable with a small laser procedure. I may add that to the docket for 2018.

Psyched to see my family this weekend! I'm so ready to go. Totally stocked up on cat food, tiny travel-size toiletries, clean laundry, cute new clothes, and fresh books to read. *Bon voyage, motherfuckers!*

Friday, December 29, 2017 | L.A. TO NEW JERSEY

Yay, vacation time! I was slightly less terrified during the flight having

Jon with me. In theory, I know a car accident is a million times more likely than a plane crash, but my stomach wraps into a knot of fear at the slightest bit of turbulence. Thankfully, the ride wasn't too bumpy, but as with every flight, I exhale an embarrassingly large sigh of relief when the plane lands safely.

We grabbed our bags and waited for a Lyft in the frigid cold. Our bodies are not accustomed to chilly weather. The ride to our hotel was quick. We checked in, and I texted my brother Rob. He was already there with his wife and kids, so we all ate dinner at the hotel restaurant, excited to start the cruise. I am so crazy about my niece and nephew. We had some mediocre food and amazing laughs and all tucked into bed. Jon and I grabbed a bottle of wine and watched a movie before nodding off.

Saturday, December 30, 2017 | NEW JERSEY PORT

PARTY TIME! Our whole motley crew met in the lobby at eight a.m. for our giant taxi, which took us to the port where we boarded the ship. As the taxi approached the port, we all marveled at how overwhelmingly huge the ship was. Like, almost *too* huge. Of course, my anxiety kicked into high gear, and I wondered how the ship would stay afloat if we encountered a tsunami. Like, if the boat tipped over, would I pull a Kate Winslet and survive by crawling onto a piece of wood? Or would I channel my inner Leonardo DiCaprio and sacrifice myself for someone I loved? Best not to think about it. Damn you, *Titanic*.

During dinner, Mom gave a very emotional, very thoughtful, toast to Jon. Everyone cried. She had written a beautiful note about how much she and Dad appreciated Jon for taking care of me during cancer. Then she told him she and Dad were going to buy him a brand new Mac computer as a thank-you. He was floored. We all were. Jon and I threw back a couple of whiskeys and went to bed, happy to be stuffed on a boat with 5,000 other people.

_____

Sunday, December 31, 2017 | SOMEWHERE IN THE ATLANTIC OCEAN

Thank you, Baby Jesus, for bringing this year to an end. Longest. Year. Ever.

2018 has to be better. It just has to be. It will be.

Today we were at sea all day. Hit the gym, then the hot tub, then the gorgeous indoor spa area at the top of the ship.

During tonight's dinner, Dad stood up and gave me a toast for being such a warrior and an inspiration during cancer. It was so unexpected, and I sobbed. *Damnit, Dad!* Jon and I were the only ones awake for the midnight countdown, so we hit one of the bars with a beautiful piano, huge plush leather couches, and a nice drink menu. The guy at the piano was a disappointment, though, because he didn't know any popular Sinatra tunes. Boo.

We each had champagne and an Old Fashioned. We watched a few episodes of *Silicon Valley* in bed and resolved to make 2018 our best year yet. As I drifted off, I silently bid farewell to the year of pandemonium and made space to welcome in a year of peace.

Goodbye, 2017. And a giant fuck you.

_____

Tuesday, January 2, 2018 | FLORIDA

Today was gray and rainy, but the family wanted to take the kids to Disney World. Jon and I stayed behind. I rationalized that my weak immune system couldn't handle rain AND thousands of coughing toddlers at a packed theme park.

Later on, we had a great family dinner. The kids were adorable in their little dressy outfits, and Anita (my brother Brian's girlfriend) is so good with them. Which is no surprise since she works in the

PICU (Pediatric Intensive Care Unit). I'm happy she fits so well with my family.

After dinner, Jon and I visited the Bionic Bar, an amazing spot where you order a cocktail on an iPad, and a robot serves you. I love technology.

We were enjoying our vodka concoctions, when, out of nowhere, I had a total fucking meltdown. I cried and cried and cried. Jon didn't ask any questions, and seeing me cry made him cry.

I apologized for making a scene as I sobbed into my cocktail. *What the fuck caused this emotional outburst?* On the surface, everything seemed fine—I finished chemo, I had my entire family around, and this was my victory vacation! But something nagged at my soul. A sense of longing with a sense of sadness. I probably didn't want to admit this (even to myself), but I think I longed to have my own children, and it hurt my heart to see Anita bonding so rapidly with my niece and nephew, while I feared that Jon will never want kids. *And that could be a deal breaker. God, that's heartbreaking to consider.*

Cancer has put an annoyingly large mirror in front of my face, forcing me to evaluate what I want out of life. And I'm not necessarily comfortable with what I see.

After about twenty minutes, I calmed down. Jon and I meandered into the cruise ship concert hall, where a cover band was playing. We bopped around on the dance floor for a few songs, attempting to erase the emotional grease I had barfed all over us. It kinda worked, and we went to bed soon thereafter. I fell asleep dissecting my breakdown and vowed to make sense of it with Bill once I get back to L.A.

Wednesday, January 3, 2018 | NASSAU, BAHAMAS

I'd been looking forward to today, because we docked at Nassau. After breakfast, a few of us de-boated and walked to the nearest beach. It was...how shall I say...kinda like Venice Beach in Los

Angeles, in that it was less pristine and exotic, and more surrounded by construction and graffiti. But it was a beach, nonetheless. We played around in the ocean and enjoyed the warm sun. Dad and I swam around and took a second to marvel that THIS was the vacation I'd been dreaming about during chemo. THIS was the moment I envisioned during those eighteen treatments of hell.

Yeah, lying in the sand is way better than lying in a bed with IVs penetrating your skin.

Thursday, January 4, 2018 | SOMEWHERE IN THE ATLANTIC OCEAN

Today we were supposed to dock at some island, but the ocean was too choppy, so the captain announced we'd be at sea all day. As well as tomorrow. And the next day.

OHMYGOD, three full days of sea time! Is now a bad time to mention I have a fear of being trapped on a boat in the middle of the ocean?

I wanted to take a crack at the giant rock climbing wall on the top deck. It was thirty-eight degrees outside, with howling winds. Not surprisingly, there were only a few people in line. Anita came with me and we exchanged looks—the wall was much higher than we'd anticipated. They strapped you into a harness so you wouldn't plummet to your death, but it was still scary. I'd been bouldering a couple of times before (which means there's no harness and the walls are much lower to the ground), but this was a whole different vibe. Anita went first, and she almost reached the top. Then it was my turn, and the first few grips were pretty easy to hang on to. But about halfway up the wall, it got a lot harder. My arms felt weak, the wind was forceful, and I stupidly looked down for a second. *OH GOD, THIS IS SCARY.* I clung to those tiny grips for dear life. I was only two grips away from the top when my hands gave out. Even though I didn't reach the top, I was still proud. As I slowly rappelled downward, I tipped my head back in laughter, and it hit one of the rocks. I yelped, and everyone below had a good chuckle.

Saturday, January 6, 2018 | SOMEWHERE IN THE ATLANTIC OCEAN

Final day at sea. I'm kinda ready to return to my cats and job hunting and my bed. And to therapy, where Bill and I can dissect the fucked up layers of my psyche that caused my meltdown. I'm sure giving Bill a run for his money.

Apparently Boston was hit with a "bomb cyclone" of snow. Is that a real thing? And do I really want to move back there? I'll need to ponder.

Our last family dinner was delicious and bittersweet. I ordered lobster. As everyone ate, I quietly observed my dad interacting with the kids, and I fought the lump in my throat. *He is such a good dad and granddad. He's kind and attentive. I want my own kid to get to know him the way I do. Fuck, I'm on the verge of another meltdown. Thank God I didn't put on mascara.*

Sunday, January 7, 2018 | NEW JERSEY

Aaaaaaaand, it's De-Boat Day. I slept like crap. Jon and I hit the buffet for bagels and sat with Mom and Dad. My heart was heavy knowing I had to say goodbye, but I'll be back in Boston soon.

I wistfully hugged every family member, and Jon and I took a Lyft to our hotel. It was absolutely frigid outside waiting for the car. Back at the hotel (same one we stayed at last week), we literally did nothing but eat and watch TV all day. I definitely felt like the world was swaying and I got queasy—I think they call it "land sickness." After lunch, we went back to bed and napped. Later we ordered room service and gorged on fries, chicken wings, and greasy sandwiches. I fell asleep with tummy gurgles and a twinge of regret. Any time I eat like this, I picture evil cancer cells growing inside my gut.

———

Monday, January 8, 2018 | NEW JERSEY TO L.A.

The flight back to L.A. wasn't too bumpy, but I was terrified of the turbulence and thought a panic attack could be on the horizon. Jon suggested we watch *Creed* to distract me. We both love boxing, so I figured we'd love the film...but I wish someone had told me that Rocky Balboa gets cancer (sorry, spoiler). He goes through chemo and loses his hair and still manages to train Adonis Creed. I was entirely too emotionally fragile for that crap. Jon and I spent the better part of two hours mopping off our eyes.

———

Tuesday, January 9, 2018

Happy to be home, but I'm having a tough time adjusting to land. This vertigo is insane. I feel dizzy, lightheaded, and I can't really think straight. (Which I love if I've been drinking...but not sober.) Such a weird feeling. I cancelled therapy, and Bill said we'd reschedule when I'm better. Jon is worried this might be the beginning of pneumonia, but Dad said I'd be coughing if that were the case. I drank water, ate soup, and prayed I didn't bring home a disease from the cruise ship.

A girl from Cedars called (referred from Sarah), and they want to feature my story on their blog. We'll do an in-person interview and photoshoot at my apartment. I'm hoping it goes well, and REALLY hoping it leads to a full-time job at Cedars as a content creator. They're coming over in a week, so I have exactly seven days to reduce the number of chins currently residing under my face.

Wednesday, January 10, 2018

Woke up every hour on the hour last night. My temperature is 98.8, which is reassuring, but between this headache and cough I'm developing, I'm paranoid about dying of pneumonia. I called my Primary Care and got an appointment for tomorrow.

I miss that feeling when you were young and felt invincible, like nothing can hurt you. This whole, *I'm gonna be killed from an ear infection* shit is for the birds. Fuckin' cancer. Took two Nyquil and tucked away for the night.

Thursday, January 11, 2018

My Primary Care assured me I don't have pneumonia or an ear infection, and the dizziness is from my ear fluid being all outta whack. Whew. She said to keep doing what I'm doing (resting, Vitamin C, fluids, soup, etc) and use saline to clean out my sinuses twice a day.

I desperately needed to get out of the house, so I hiked with Kara. I felt dizzy but managed to trudge up Runyon Canyon at a good pace. Saturday is supposed to be our nine-mile marathon training run, and despite feeling that I should refrain, I told her I'd do it.

Whatever, I can rest when I'm dead.

Saturday, January 13, 2018

OK, I probably should have rested. The run was a massive struggle, and I kept fighting the urge to quit. I was slow, sluggish, and off-balance. But I did it.

Now that we're into a fresh year, I've been thinking about career and financial goals. I'm really into making lists, so I'm gonna come up with eighteen goals for 2018. Time to start visualizing and manifesting!

1. Finish my children's book.
2. Self-publish cancer diary.
3. Complete L.A. marathon.
4. Complete a Tough Mudder.
5. Meditate daily.
6. Find a yoga studio and go weekly, or bi-weekly.
7. Expand my cooking horizons beyond veggie burgers and zucchini noodles.
8. Knock out ten pull-ups at once.
9. Make more lists.
10. Eat more cheese.
11. Write at least two blog posts a month.
12. Finish the short story that I started writing in college.
13. Go back to Sedona.
14. Learn how to apply a flawless, full face of makeup.
15. Pay off credit card balance, add to 401(k), build up savings account.
16. Bake a cake without fucking it up.
17. Reach goal weight of 140 with lots of muscle.
18. STOP STRESSING SO FUCKING MUCH ABOUT EVERYTHING. (Obviously the most challenging, and I'm not even sure this is possible.)

Monday, January 15, 2018

Realized I haven't weighed myself in a while, so I apprehensively stepped on the scale. 149. Not too mad at that. After a week of nonstop drinking during the cruise, I thought the damage would be worse. I don't even want to lose much more weight—maybe ten pounds. I'm more interested in tightening and increasing my strength. The stronger I get, the easier my double mastectomy will be.

I'm nervous about the Cedars photoshoot tomorrow. Logically, I know it'll go smoothly, but I hate being in front of the camera. And I get anxious when people put me on the spot. Plus, I'm still bloated from the cruise, so I'm hoping Cedars has a Photoshop wizard that can retouch me into a dazzling, thin, cancer-free goddess.

Tuesday, January 16, 2018

Eep! It's time for my closeup, Mr. DeMille. I cleaned, then re-cleaned my apartment. Picked out a cute sleeveless black top and threw on some makeup (to the best of my ability). For some reason, my skin decided to unleash a giant blemish on the middle of my nose—but not one of those little demure blemishes you can mask with makeup. No, it was one of those horrendous weird rashes that no amount of concealer will hide. I literally slathered on eight layers of cover-up, and it did nothing. Oh well. I compensated by putting on eight layers of dark eyeliner. Hopefully that will draw the attention away from the red honker on my schnauze.

The Cedars crew showed up a few minutes early, and they were super sweet. I felt like I was posing for my high school senior portraits most of the time, but we got some shots in my pool area that looked great. We casually talked about my diagnosis and the chemo treatments. They asked me to visit their studio next week for another shoot, this time with my costumes and wigs, and we'd do the official interview then. Whew! That ought to be enough time for Kimmy-The-Red-Nosed-Reindeer to return to normal.

Thursday, January 18, 2018

Went to therapy and cried for forty-five minutes. I don't think Bill expected the emotional tsunami I let loose, but I hadn't seen him in three weeks, and I had to empty my mental garbage. Honestly,

I barely remember what we talked about, but I felt twenty pounds lighter walking back to my car.

I received a really sad text from Tina, my bestie from high school, to tell me her mom passed away. So devastated for her. The funeral is next Friday, so I'll fly in the day before and stay for a week. I'm glad I'll get to see family and friends, but I wish it were under different circumstances. And God, I truly wish there were something I could do to ease Tina's pain. Life is so unfair sometimes.

Monday, January 22, 2018

Strike a pose! It's Cedars picture day. I packed a couple of outfits, threw on some hastily-applied makeup, and headed to the studio. The nerves in my belly thrashed around, and my palms were sweaty. I'm thrilled for the opportunity to share my story, but I'll never get over my fear of being in front of the camera.

Why didn't I put whiskey in my coffee?

Al, the photographer, did his best to calm me down. He put on some music and set up the lighting while I arranged my wigs on a table. I was shaking for the first several photos, but Al joked around and eventually I relaxed.

The content writer, Canon, came in and we did my interview. It was casual and chill, just like talking to a friend. We got off-topic a couple of times and had some giggles. I really like her and wistfully thought about how cool it'd be to join her team.

You haven't seen the last of me, Cedars. I shall find a way to infiltrate your staff and create awesome content for you. <insert maniacal laughter>

Went home and wiped off my makeup (which had smudged all over my face by that point). I can't wait to read the blog! It'll be such an honor to see my photo on the Cedars website, among fellow cancer survivors and other heroes. *Hey, maybe cancer will be my ticket to stardom?*

Tuesday, January 23, 2018

Had a great solo session in therapy. We talked about things that totally caught me off guard. Bill kept challenging me and got me to think about why I constantly seek other people's approval. Why I want everyone to like me. Why I want everyone to think I'm nice and funny and sweet and cool. I concluded that I want those things because I'm super fucking insecure.

"OK. Why do you think you're so insecure?"

I paused. I had no fucking clue.

"Were you mistreated by anyone when you were younger?"

No, I had the best childhood ever. My parents were (and still are) saints. I had great friends. But there was one chick in high school who tormented me and called me names and poured soda down my back during an assembly. *What a bitch. I forgot how much that hurt my feelings.*

"OK. Well, do you think it's possible you have this need to be well-liked as a defense mechanism? Because if people like you, they won't hurt you."

Woh.

Wednesday, January 24, 2018

Packed for Boston and went for a jog. Huffed and puffed the whole way, and wondered why I agreed to run a marathon.

Went to Cedars to meet with The Breast Whisperer Dr. Dang. She said my MRI looked fine, and there's absolutely no cancer in my chest. She did a quick exam and, thankfully, everything felt normal.

"Yay! So now, on to the important stuff—my boob job!"

Dr. Dang smiled. She explained that during the double mastectomy, she will remove all my breast tissue. The reconstructive surgeon (whom I'll soon meet) will insert either tissue expanders or implants. Apparently the tissue expanders will be more painful and more of a pain in the ass, but they give my skin time to heal and readjust before shoving in permanent implants.

Then there's the question of what to do with my nipples. Some women are unable to keep theirs, due to sagging issues from aging or having children. Dr. Dang said mine are fine, so I could keep them, but then there's a small layer of tissue that remains, and it could be a potential place for cancer to grow. If we remove the nipples, we could either reconstruct them from my own skin, or do a 3D tattoo. These two options can potentially lower the risk of cancer developing, since there's no layer of tissue there, but might be less aesthetic. We also have to consider whether the implant would go over or under the muscle. Ugh. I'll know once I meet with the plastic surgeon, but I felt deflated after hearing how complicated this could get.

All I know is, #NippleLivesMatter. Ooooh, that'd make an excellent bumper sticker.

Thursday, January 25, 2018 | L.A. TO BOSTON

Couldn't sleep well and woke up at four a.m. before my alarm went off. Super apprehensive and sad about the memorial service.

Oh, and BTW, I HATE flying.

Took an Ativan to calm down and it helped. Virgin stopped updating their TV and movie offerings, so I watched *Snatched* for the fifth time. Also, I brought my teddy bear for comfort, and I think the guy one row over was judging me.

After landing, I grabbed a Lyft to Mom & Dad's house, and I asked the driver to stop for coffee because I needed caffeine. Thankfully he didn't mind (or at least acted like he didn't), and I slurped down the eighty-ounce almond coffee before I got out of the car. Mom put fresh roses in my room and clean white folded towels in the bathroom. Yay to Hotel Tronic! She said my hair looks thick and healthy.

I took ZzzQuil and CBD oil and crawled into bed around midnight. It'll be sad to say goodbye to Tina's mom tomorrow, but I'm glad I could be here.

———————

Friday, January 26, 2018 | BOSTON

Guh. I knew today would be tough. But the memorial service (held at a Lutheran church) was beautiful, and felt like the right way to remember Tina's mom. I mostly held it together, but I was *wrecked* at something Tina's dad said. He talked about true love and what it meant. In the weeks and months leading up to his wife's passing, he would lie next to her, sleep next to her, and attend to her every need. And as tough as it was to be in his position, that's what you do for someone you love. That's what unconditional love is. You don't even give it a second thought or question it.

Sniff. Sob. Sniff. Sob. Why didn't I bring more tissues?!

Afterwards, everyone had lunch at a nearby country club and socialized. I got to talk with Tina's dad and brother, which was nice. And I caught up with Sue, whom I hadn't seen in eighteen years. (She used to run cross-country with me and Tina. Sue is hilariously goofy—we'd imitate *Sesame Street* characters, but say horribly crude and perverted things in Grover or Elmo's voice to distract ourselves from how much we hated running.)

I'll admit I'm crazy jealous of her life now. She's a successful real estate agent with a beautiful house in a beautiful town with three gorgeous kids and a doting husband. And here I am, unemployed, living alone in a one bedroom apartment with cracked walls, coming off a cancer battle with a huge scar on my stomach, sad short choppy hair, bags under my eyes, and riddled with anxiety and resentment. I know you're not supposed to compare yourself to other people, but....

I came home, took a hot shower, and decided to go to Tina's since they were having family over. Mom and I baked a decadent coffee cake for me to bring. (OK, fine, Mom baked it and I watched her. OK fine, Mom baked it and I watched TV. But she enjoys baking and I would have just gotten in the way.)

Tina's brother, dad, husband, and a few relatives were eating and drinking wine, and I was happily surprised at how upbeat the vibe was. Tina and I got to catch up and crack a lot of jokes. But there was still a heaviness in the air and I know we all felt the loss like an invisible punch to the gut.

God, family really is the most important thing. I need to make sure I acknowledge that every single day from now on.

Saturday, January 27, 2018 | BOSTON

Oh, right, the marathon is coming up. I should probably go for a run. But it's twenty-eight degrees out. Boo.

Forced myself to jog, and Rob brought his kids over. I wrestled around with my niece and nephew, and took a second to appreciate them. I can't believe I didn't want kids. Anika is such a sweet, beautiful, smart little girl. I would do anything to raise a daughter like her. And Kiran is such a trip, too. He's hyper and hilarious, and it truly brings me joy to see how much my parents love their grandkids.

Also, I just realized that it's been exactly one year since I began this crazy journey.

It seems surreal. In the last twelve months, I lost my job, was diagnosed with Stage Three ovarian cancer, endured eighteen chemo sessions, had my ovaries removed, had my uterus removed, had my spleen removed, lost thirty pounds, gained eight pounds back, had my cat diagnosed with cancer, got him through nine chemo sessions, went to Sedona, discovered my love of meditation, began training for my fifth marathon, began seeing a therapist, got signed

168 I DEAR DIARY

by a literary agent, made some incredible new friends, shaved my head (several times), got a huge new tattoo, and learned a whole lot about myself. Sheesh. What a year.

So, where do I go from here?

Well, with a double mastectomy hanging in the rafters, I feel like I can't totally move past this chapter of my life. And I've got a million questions about the future of my relationship, job situation, health, and everything else.

Will Jon and I end up together? With all my physical scars, emotional baggage, and inability to have children, am I even marriage material? When will I get a full-time job? Do I even want a full-time job? Should I just launch my own company? Will I ever get a cancer recurrence? When will my breast surgery be? Should I get giant implants, or sensibly-sized ones? Should I move back to Boston? What kind of candy should I binge on right now?

Basically, I have no clue what's next. But that's alright—I've realized it's totally OK not to have the answers. Because honestly, no one does. And now I've got a second chance at life, so I'm determined to make the most of it and grab life by the balls—while making sure my ass doesn't look too fat.

Xoxo

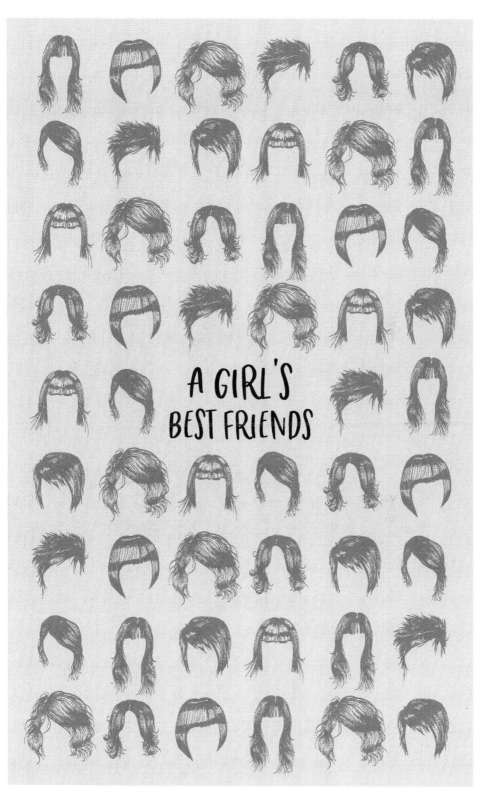

A GIRL'S
BEST FRIENDS

AUTHOR'S NOTE

WOW, YOU'RE STILL READING? And you still care what I have to say? You need more hobbies. Or maybe you're just bored, waiting for new episodes of *The Walking Dead*. Either way, thanks for sticking with me 'til the end.

You know how people say hindsight is 20/20? Mine's probably blurrier, but maybe that's the whiskey. Even though I've put the worst behind me, I continue to struggle. I attend therapy once a week. I have good days and bad days. And certain things can trigger me at the drop of a hat. But rather than focus on everything that cancer *took* from me, I've flipped the script, and I'm grateful for what it *gave* me.

Enduring the cancer shit storm awakened a dormant side of my psyche.

I think of it as a "reintroduction to my life."

And not to sound like a bullshit self-help book from the bargain bin at Barnes & Noble, but perspective really is everything. My post-cancer days are sprinkled with a deep collection of epiphanies that have allowed me to live a better, fuller life.

If you haven't already, now would be a great time to get popcorn.

Go ahead, I'll wait. My favorite is White Cheddar Skinny Pop.

You good now? OK let's do this. May I present Kim's Official Cancer Takeaways:

(By the way, none of these ideologies were particularly earth-shattering—I'd heard them all at one point or another—but as a direct result of my ordeal, they became clear and meaningful and suddenly made a fuck-ton of sense.)

1) The important stuff is the intangible stuff.

We live in a society where we're taught to want things: cars, houses, the new iPhone, a Dyson vacuum. (Admittedly, I'm guilty of that last one—I really enjoy cleaning, OK?) And we're bombarded with this message everywhere: commercials, TV, movies, billboards, magazines, and the digital stratosphere.

Even social media feeds into the more, more, more mentality—just scroll through Facebook and Instagram, and you're greeted with a pile of #humblebrags about those ugly new Kanye shoes or your cousin's dope BMW. And *voila*, a place that was conceived to foster connection ends up dividing us between those who have this stuff and those who don't.

It's easy to let the years slip by in a revolving door of wanting stuff. I certainly did. Then I got a giant bitch-slap from the Universe and my outlook did a complete 180. When you're faced with your own mortality in a very real way, the insignificant stuff flakes away until you're left in a world where material things lose every ounce of value.

The intangible stuff, the stuff that really matters, is the stuff you can't hold in your hands. But you hold it in your heart. In your soul. In your memories.

Family. Friendship. Love. Health. Community. These are your greatest assets. They are beautiful and invaluable, and you can't take them for granted. They are the things that truly make us whole, and sadly, a lot of people don't appreciate them until they're gone.

As you get older and reflect back on your life, what do you think you'll remember? Will it be the material stuff or the intangible stuff? Will it be all the crap you amassed, or will it be your relationships?

(But for real, if anyone wants to send me a Dyson vacuum, that would be super awesome.)

2) Don't "tomorrow" yourself to death.

I'll start eating healthy tomorrow. I'll apply for my dream job tomorrow. I'll get my shit together tomorrow. I'll work toward the life I want tomorrow.

Sound familiar? Many of my goals were "tomorrow-ed" away over the years until they either fell off the radar or I moved them into "today."

Now I look back and think, *What the hell was I waiting for?*

Time is a precious commodity. It doesn't discriminate. You can't buy more of it. If you waste it, you're not gonna get it back.

Cancer lit a huge proverbial fire under my ass, and lemme tell you, this tush is burning (and not in the gross food-poisoning-toilet way). As I waded through my post-cancer cognitive catastrophe, I contemplated everything on my Bucket List. What would I do if I weren't scared or financially-strapped? What if I didn't let the uncertainty and anxiety and noise in my head make the rules? I would set out to cross those missions off the list, one by one.

And really, if I waited around to make more money or gain a slew of self-assurance, I could easily die inside a casket of tomorrows. Why should I wait? There will never be a "good" time to chase my dreams. These fictitious barriers holding me back are just that-useless figments of my overactive imagination.

So I said FUCK IT. I knocked out a book. I started a sequel. I began a super secret side project that you'll hear about in the near future. I learned how to cook. I learned how to walk in high heels without breaking an ankle. I stopped procrastinating and started everything I thought I couldn't.

The moral of the story? Quit. Fucking. Waiting.

3) Stop the "I'll be happy when…" gibberish.

Of all my toxic thought patterns (and trust me, there are plenty), this was the hardest to move past.

I think we all get caught up in the "milestones mindset" at some point. It's so easy to pin your happiness on a yet-to-be-achieved-landmark. *I'll be happy when I get married. When I have 2.5 kids. Get a dog. And score my dream job.*

I've done this my entire life. I can remember thinking I'd be happy once I turned thirteen, then once I turned sixteen, then once I started college, then once I graduated college, and so on and so on.

But the problem is you'll never be happy. The mileposts always move to something else.

During my ordeal, I kept thinking I'd be happy after the cancer was removed from my body. And I did feel relief once I bid farewell to those devious tumors, but I didn't magically hop a train into Happyville. Because the milepost moved. My post-cancer happiness suddenly depended on a whole new set of stipulations.

It took me many months and dozens of therapy sessions to grasp the antidote. An answer so simple, one that I'd heard so many times, but could never truly comprehend until I'd trudged through the depths of Hades.

Be. Happy. Now.

Whaaat? How was I supposed to be happy and fulfilled with a frail body, battered soul, and giant list of unchecked accomplishments? Easy: just decide to be.

See, the more we reach outward for things to make us happy, the more we should reach within. Sure, it's OK to want things for your life, but those things shouldn't dictate your happiness or hold it hostage.

Once I realized that I can be happy now, and that I already have tons to be grateful for, wouldn't ya know it—those nagging mileposts started to disintegrate, and I enjoyed life a lot more. Truthfully, there are still days I grapple with this (hey, I'm only human), but the more I detach my happiness from unattained experiences, the more content I feel—exactly as I am.

So, do yourself a favor and quit moving the milestones. Or even better—destroy them.

4) Believe in yourself.

I admit, this sounds like a corny poster from your seventh grade homeroom. Go ahead and roll your eyes. But hear me out.

As a writer, marketer, and content creator, I'm my own biggest critic. I'm an expert at convincing myself that everything I do is crap. My default mode is, *I sound dumb. No one will care. People will judge me or make fun of me. Oh, sure I'm writing a book, but no one's gonna read it. Why even bother promoting it if it's gonna be forgotten in a week?*

You know that quote, "Whether you think you can or cannot, you're right"? Well, if you think you suck and your work is shit, you'll find yourself in the midst of a self-fulfilling prophecy.

I had unknowingly limited myself. Kept myself in a little box. Held myself down, thinking I'm not capable, or I don't deserve success. But why? Why did I care what other people thought? Why did I need other people to validate me and my work? Why didn't I set ambitious goals?

I blame a crippling sense of insecurity. Many years ago, a former boss had the gall to tell me my writing sucked. (He didn't actually use the word "suck" but you get the idea.) I was crushed. How could I possibly make a career out of writing and content creation if this guy said I couldn't?

I should have thanked him for the motivation.

But I believed him at the time, and it took years to undo the self-doubt he smeared all over me. Slowly, through tons of encouragement and support, I cautiously collected tidbits of confidence, and my cancer experience ended up solidifying a sense of self-certainty.

Now I know I can do whatever I want. I can set lofty goals and accomplish them. I can reach for the stars. And so can you. (Also, to play devil's advocate for a second—I think it's important to set goals, but not let your happiness DEPEND on those goals. By eliminating the milestone mindset, your fulfillment isn't contingent upon your accomplishments, but it's healthy to work toward your aspirations.)

So, believe in yourself! If you don't, no one else will.

5) Fear can be really powerful—but so can hope.

As humans, fear developed as a natural reaction to keep us safe from danger, and it's still useful in the right setting. But I think we've overdeveloped this safety mechanism, and it materializes in the wrong places.

Fear prevents us from living. From moving forward. From taking risks and making decisions. It's designed to hold us back. Prime example: back in 2014, I worked at a production company that gravely mistreated and underpaid its employees. Everyone on my team felt miserable, and one by one, people quit. I stayed there, unhappy and defeated, for much longer than I should have—because I was scared to leave. What if I couldn't find another job? What if I spent the next two years hunting for a new opportunity but no one hires me and I'll have to drain my 401(k) and eat non-organic food and buy the cheap cat food for my babies but they develop kidney stones because I couldn't afford the high-end kitty chow?

I like to think back to my childhood. Fear never even entered my mind—I rode my bike without worrying about falling, I ran through the woods without worrying about kidnappers, and I took candy from strangers at Halloween without worrying about poison. (Well, not really, but you get my point.)

Then I grew up, became scared of everything, got cancer, and became even more scared of everything. *What if the cancer returns? When's the huge L.A. earthquake gonna happen? Will I ever get my shit together in my career? What if this book is a failure? What if it's not?*

After tons of therapy and self-reflection (thanks, Bill!), I eventually understood that it's counterproductive to live life through a fear-colored filter. Wanna know what's better? Approaching life from a place of hope.

When you have hope, you feel like you can do anything. OK, in reality, no one can do everything (unless you're Beyoncé), but hope is a portal to possibilities, opportunities, and self-worth. It melts away the doubt. It lets you explore, be curious, and experience a broader range of existence.

I'm hopeful that I kicked cancer. That I'll stay healthy. That I'll lead a long fulfilling life and crush my goals.

Fear holds you back. Hope moves you forward. The choice is yours.

6) Find your purpose.

I know, I know, can I stop with the clichés already?

Have you ever wondered what the purpose of life is? Why we're here? What we're supposed to do with our time on Earth?

In my pre-cancer days, I didn't give this much thought. I just wanted to have as much fun as possible. But when the Ovarian Cancer Grim Reaper suddenly showed up, I started asking myself a slew of questions:

What am I doing here? What motivates me to get up in the morning? What have I accomplished? What do I want to accomplish?

I think we all have a purpose (whether we realize it or not). It may be as simple as being a mom or a dad. Or as arduous as solving the climate crisis. We've all been blessed with a chance to do something special with our time—why waste that?

For months, I let these thoughts simmer in the back burner of my brain. I didn't come to any quick conclusions, but I kept an open mind and discussed this with my therapist, brothers, and friends. It slowly became clear that I wanted to help people in some way, to give back to my community, to contribute to humanity. What would that look like? I wasn't sure, but those elements of purpose felt good to me.

After spending a year obsessing over my health, my looks, and my mental state, it felt amazing to look outside myself and ponder how I could help other people. It was liberating. And even though this portion of my life is still a work in progress, I see the significance at looking inside myself. Opening my mind. Getting curious. Asking questions—to myself, and to others. Making new discoveries. Finding the things that push me forward and make me a better person.

What drives you? What's your purpose?

7) It's OK to feel like shit sometimes.
Lots of people ask how I was able to stay so upbeat and optimistic during cancer. I've actually wondered the same thing, and I think it's a multi-pronged answer.

First, I've always been that way. Cheeriness is part of my DNA. (Thanks, Mom!) And for that, I'm grateful—I truly believe that my temperament played a big role in my recovery. My natural enthusiasm left me better equipped to handle all the shit thrown my way, and my energy level merely decreased from insanely hyperactive to normal.

Second, my prognosis made it easier to retain a sunny outlook. After the initial shock of the diagnosis wore off, I started to understand that eventually I would be OK. The situation morphed from,

OMG I'm gonna die to *Alright, this is atrocious but it's only temporary.* If my Rockstar Cancer Ninja Dr. Li had told me on that fateful afternoon it was Stage Four and I only had a few months to live, do you think I would have been so sprightly? No way.

So, the reason is partially inherent, partially circumstantial. Now, having said that, things got darker than I'd anticipated—the highs were higher than expected, but the lows were lower.

There were days I felt so sick, so depressed, so battered and beat down, I honestly wondered if I'd ever feel joy again. Then I'd scold myself for giving in to the negativity, thinking I had a responsibility to remain positive. Even my social media posts during that time were peppered with smiles, jokes, and happy anecdotes.

But why? Why couldn't I admit that I felt despondent, that I spent days crying and crying and crying? Why did I feel obligated to put on a brave face? Probably because my jovial default mode was so different than the misery I experienced. This level of gloom was new and uncomfortable.

Looking back, I wish I would have recognized that it's OK to feel like absolute shit. I tried to fight it, instead of giving into it and letting myself feel awful. (Side note: I don't think that crying and feeling despondent are classified as "giving in" to the grief—they were merely visceral reactions to the agony, but I didn't let those moments of temporary darkness turn into weeks, or months, of sadness.) I've since realized that it's perfectly healthy, even constructive, to sit in those tortured moments (as long as you don't stay there for an extended period of time). Those occasions can teach us a whole lot about ourselves.

Next time you get into that headspace, I invite you to take a moment and reflect. Rather than bury it, push back against it, or release it, try hitting the pause button and see what you can learn from it. Because I think the most substantial growth we do as humans stems from exactly that.

8) Never stop evolving.

Right in the middle of chemo treatments, I remember seeing a cool piece of graffiti in Hollywood from my favorite street artist, WRDSMTH—a spray painted typewriter that said, 'Your life is under construction. Expect delays."

I nodded in agreement, contemplating how much my life had stopped dead in its tracks because of cancer. I was definitely under construction. Cancer broke me. I lived each day among a figurative pile of rubble, pissed that my body, my psyche, my entire life just got torn down.

Later on, I thought about the concept of construction—you break something down and demolish it into a million little pieces. But then something great happens—you rebuild something new, something better. The same could be said about me. Cancer demolished me, but I got rebuilt. Restored into something new, something better, something stronger.

The new Kim ("Kim 2.0") is now set on a foundation of regrowth and mended mentalities. And that new foundation set into motion a new process of evolution. One where I'm exploring my spirituality, I'm constantly striving to be the best version of myself, I'm trying new things, and I'm taking new risks. I'm like an Apple app—I have an annoying amount of updates.

With evolution, there's always room for growth and discovery; wouldn't life be boring if we stayed exactly the same? I think it's arrogant to believe that you know everything, that there's nothing else to learn, that change isn't necessary.

Becoming a better version of yourself is exciting. It's a world of prospects, a place where potential is right at your fingertips. But change can also be painful during the "life under construction" phase. I say, go grab one of those yellow safety helmets and a bag of White Cheddar Skinny Pop. Brace yourself.

"Kim 3.0" is right around the corner. And if we're lucky, she'll pass "You 2.0" along the way.

In conclusion, dear reader, I hope you never experience the depths of pain, heartaches, and headaches that accompany a cancer diagnosis, but if you do, please know you're not alone. There's a bevy of us beauties who have kicked cancer's ass, and we're waiting in the wings to hug you, comfort you, and welcome you to the club. Sure, it's a membership you never wanted, but I promise even the darkest experiences can unlock a better, happier version of you. (And maybe a smaller ass.)

ACKNOWLEDGMENTS

IT TAKES A VILLAGE to beat cancer. It also takes one to publish a book. Without these incredible humans, neither scenario would have happened.

Jon Rygiewicz (Ryg, Rygger, Rygglesbee, Noodle, Doodle, Boodle, Chester Puppercup), for sticking by my side throughout the hardest time of our lives. You are my rock.

Freddy Tran Nager, for your endless encouragement, inspiration, wit, proofreading, guidance, friendship, and invaluable role as my mentor.

Rachel Beller, for your nutrition mastery, astute advice, infinite kindness, and gaggle of giggles we've shared.

John DeDakis, for your brilliant editing insights, and suggestion to include you in the Acknowledgments.

Bill Benson, for mopping up my psychological wreckage, and showing me I can reach for the stars.

The amazing Cedars Sinai nurses, for always making me laugh during chemo: Angela Schleuniger, Casey Vastano, AJ Kiefer, Cindy Kim, and Michelle Marie.

The Cedars Sinai Content/ Community/ Social Media teams, for always letting me share my story: Sarah Vexelman, Arielle Morrison

Laufman, Katie Rosenblum, Canan Tasci, Valerie Phil.

Chris Cagurangan, for that special napkin and your lunchtime love.

L.J. Amaral, for your east coast sass and dietary dopeness.

Corina Hernandez, my Angelic Nurse Practitioner, for your smiles and pushing me through treatment when I felt like puking and giving up.

Dr. Andrew Li, my Rockstar Cancer Ninja, for literally saving my life and holding my hand the entire way, just like you promised.

Rob and Brian, for being the best brothers in the world, and showing me what it means to be a role model.

And Mom and Dad, for the unconditional love and support, without which I would've surely crumbled. We did it. I love you forever.